SECRETS OF HOMOEOPATHY

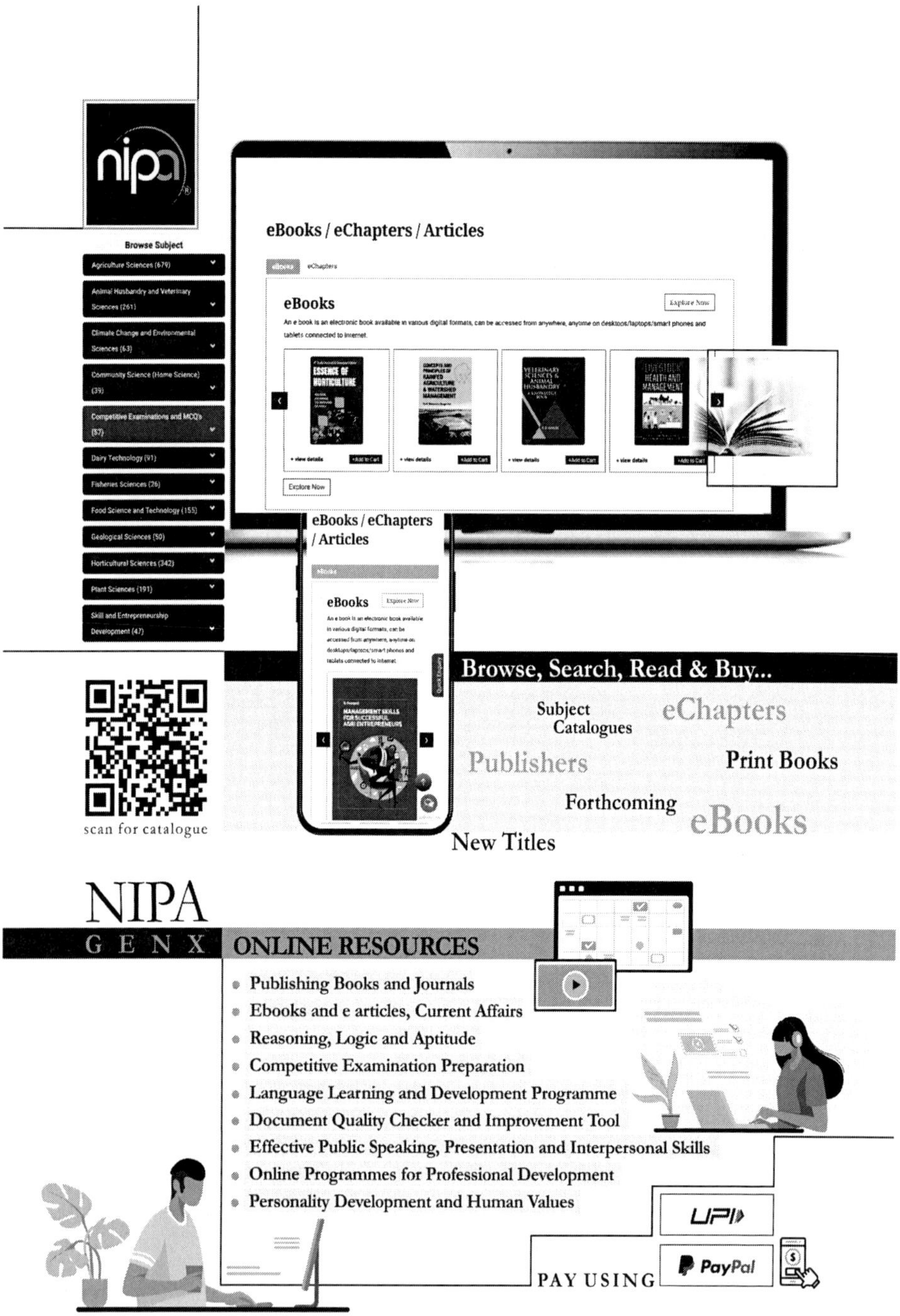
nipa
Browse Subject
Agriculture Sciences (679)
Animal Husbandry and Veterinary Sciences (261)
Climate Change and Environmental Sciences (63)
Community Science (Home Science) (39)
Competitive Examinations and MCQ's (57)
Dairy Technology (91)
Fisheries Sciences (26)
Food Science and Technology (155)
Geological Sciences (50)
Horticultural Sciences (342)
Plant Sciences (191)
Skill and Entrepreneurship Development (47)
eBooks / eChapters / Articles
eBooks
Explore Now
An e book is an electronic book available in various digital formats, can be accessed from anywhere, anytime on desktops/laptops/smart phones and tablets connected to internet.
Explore Now
scan for catalogue
Browse, Search, Read & Buy...
Subject Catalogues
eChapters
Publishers
Print Books
Forthcoming
eBooks
New Titles
NIPA
GENX
ONLINE RESOURCES
Publishing Books and Journals
Ebooks and e articles, Current Affairs
Reasoning, Logic and Aptitude
Competitive Examination Preparation
Language Learning and Development Programme
Document Quality Checker and Improvement Tool
Effective Public Speaking, Presentation and Interpersonal Skills
Online Programmes for Professional Development
Personality Development and Human Values
PAY USING
UPI
PayPal

SECRETS OF HOMOEOPATHY

Author

Dr. RITU JAIN

B.H.M.S

Homoeopathic Medical College and Hospital

Sector - 26, Chandigarh

2007

New India Publishing Agency

Pitam Pura, New Delhi- 110 088

Published by
Sumit Pal Jain *for*
New India Publishing Agency
101, Vikas Surya Plaza, CU Block, L.S.C. Mkt.,
Pitam Pura, New Delhi- 110 088, (India)
Phone: 011-27341717, Fax: 011-27341616
E-mail: newindiapublishingagency@gmail.com
Web: www.bookfactoryindia.com

Typeset at: Laxmi Art Creations, Delhi and Printed at: Jai Bharat Printing Press, Delhi

"I Treat He Cures"

Member :
Council of Homoeopathic System of Medicine (U.T.) Chandigarh

Authorised Medical Attendent :
Central Govt. Employees Indian Airlines, & O.C.F.

Dr. Sandeep Puri
D.H.M.S.
Asstt. Professor & Sr. Medical Officer
Homoeopathic Medical College & Hospital, Sector-26, Chandigarh

Resi. Cum Clinic : Kothi No. 3051, Sector-40-D, Chandigarh • College : 781760; Clinic : 692204; Resi. : 687707

Foreword

Its my pleasure to foreword a book titled **"Secrets of Homoeopathy"** compiled by Dr. Ritu Jain an ardent and intelligent product of Homoeopathic Medical College and Hospital, Sector-26, Chandigarh. Her talent is reflected in this in this book and hence makes it valuable.

This book gives a clear understanding to the learners and correct idea about practical aspecs of Homoeopathy.

A remarkable progress has taken place in the field of Homoeopathy, especially during last few decades. I believe that this book would make its own contribution towards the strengthening the Homoeopathic System of Medicine. Rapid advancement in the field of Homoeopathy would surely and largely contribute in making Homoeopathic System the first line of treatment.

I am sure that Homoeo fraternity will accept this work with pleasure and gratitude. I gladly recommend this book to the profession.

Dr. SANDEEP PURI
Asstt. Prof. and Senior Medical Officer
Deptt. of Materia Medica
Homoeopathic Medical College and Hospital
Sector-26, Chandigarh

Preface

From the days of studies in homoeopathy I was in search of a good and simple book for the beginners but I could not get any book to satiate my requirement. This thing had been haunting my mind since then. My idea began to mature after I passed my degree from Homoeopathic Medical College, Chandigarh. During my college days, my teachers helped me to reach to the flash point. My parents had been of immense help in fully maturing my idea. In this way, the total environment upto the time contributed in the writing and preparation of this book. So I earnestly hope that the book in the present form will prove to be a boon to the new students as well as to the beginners. The language has been kept simple so as to be understood by any body and every body.

In one compact volume I have tried to introduce the reader to the system of homoeopathic healing, how it originated, what are the scientific theories underlying it and what are its advantages in terms of healing of disease and cost of treatment. In the part on materia medica a number of carefully chosen drugs have been discussed in detail. I hope that these chapters would provide a rewarding experience to the readers of this book.

While preparing this book, I have taken help from works of pioneer such as Dr. Samuel Heinemann, Dr. C. Hering, Dr. T.F. Allen, Dr. J.T. Kent. I hope that the **"Secrets of Homoeopathy"** would be used and referred to in every home. I also hope that this book be of immense advantage to students of homoeopathy.

The work has been undertaken to supply the practioners of homoeopathic medicine with reliable, practical and condensed indications for the more important remedies in disease. It is devoted to homoeopathy and from works on materia medica.

In an effort of this kind it is inevitable that some errors of omission and commission, are liable to creep in. nevertheless, scope for further improvement remains and I would welcome suggestions to this end both from teachers and students.

I am greatly thankful to my father Sh. J. P. Jain, my cousin brother Mr. J. R. Jain, all my family members and the publishers for showing this book the light of the day.

Dr. RITU JAIN
B.H.M.S
Homoeopathic Medical College & Hospital
Sector - 26, Chandigarh

CONTENTS

PART- III : HOMOEOPATHIC MATERIA MEDICA

□□□

PART – I

AN INTRODUCTION

CHAPTER 1

History of Homoeopathy

The homoeopathic system of medicine is one of the finest systems of cure available in the world. It achieves in totality the ideal laid down by its founder, Dr. Samuel Hahnemann:

"The highest ideal of cure is rapid, gentle and permanent restoration of the health, or removal and annihilation of the disease in its whole extent, in the shortest, most reliable, and most harmless way, on easily comprehensible principles".

In homoeopathy, not a single drug is used without knowing its effect on healthy human beings. Hence there is no shooting in the dark. The system operates, by and large, without laboratory tests and other expensive means of diagnosis, which are being used when not needed and that too, unfortunately on patients who can hardly afford the expenses.

Cost wise, there is no medical system in the world, which is as inexpensive as homoeopathy. No patient who requires a speedy cure without side effects can ignore homoeopathy; no doctor who has nothing but the good of his patient at heart can overlook the utility and effectiveness of homoeopathy and no Government which has to balance its budget can afford not to use homoeopathy in hospitals and other institutions run for the health and care of the sick and thus it is the most *cost effective treatment.*

The discovery of homoeopathic system of medicine makes a fascinating story.

Dr. Samuel Christian Friedrich Hahnemann (born: April 11, 1755; died: July 2, 1843), a German physician was practicing as an allopath when he made the principles of homoeopathy. He was totally dissatisfied with the present modes of medical diagnosis and treatment. He was agitated because drugs were used on patients without anyone understanding their true effect on the human mind and body. He realized the insufficiency of medical science and of the therapeutic methods of those days.

Dr. Samuel Hahnemann was a sincere seeker of truth. He was not ready to believe in the existing theories regarding the effect of drugs on the human body simply because medical men had believed in them for ages. For example it was known that Peruvian bark was effective because it had a tonic effect on the stomach.

Dr. Hahnemann found that there was no proof that this particular medicine had a tonic effect on the stomach or that it was for this reason that it could be used for intermittent fevers. Similarly for other drugs used for medicinal purposes, nothing was known about their effects on human beings and role played by them individually in the treatment of disease. Dr. Hahnemann found the well-established system illogical and unprovable. The present method of healing was based on the principle of 'Contrasis Contrasis' that is healing opposites by opposites.

Dr. Hahnemann noted that laxatives, acidity with alkalis and chronic pain with painkillers could not cure constipation. He observed that in all such cases, whatever relief was experienced in the first instance was wiped out by recurrence of the malady.

Dr. Hahnemann started, as an experiment in 1790, to test China, a drug made from Peruvian bark on himself and found that he could make himself sick by taking, twice a day, four drams on the medicine in pure form. The genius that he was, he noted that dozen of symptoms of maladies, the cure of which China was associated with were produced in his body. He wrote, " I took by way of experimentation, twice a day, 4 drams of good china. My feet, finger ends, etc. at first became cold; I grew languid and drowsy; then my heart began to palpate, and my pulse grew hard and small; intolerable anxiety, trembling, prostration throughout all my limbs; then pulsation, in the head, redness of my cheeks, thirst, and in short, all these symptoms which are ordinarily characteristic of intermittent fever, made their appearance, one after the other, yet without the actual rigor. Briefly, even those symptoms which are of regular occurrence and especially characteristic – as the stupidity of man, the kind of rigidity in all the limbs, but above all the numb, disagreeable sensation, which seems to have its seat in the periosteum, over every bone in the body – all these made their appearances. This paroxysms lasted two or three hours each day and recurred if I repeated this dose, not otherwise; I discontinued it, and was in good health."

Dr. Hahnemann found that the mental and physical symptoms produced in him corresponded exactly with the symptoms of the disease for which the doctors were prescribing China. He himself had cured such symptoms with china. It could no longer be said that Peruvian bark cured intermittent chill and fever because it was a bitter or an astringent drug. China cures certain symptoms of chill and fever because it produces the same symptoms of chill and fever in a healthy person. He thus formulated the law of 'Similia Similibus Curentur' or like cures like.' He came to the conclusion that a drug, which could, through excessive administration, produce certain symptoms of the body and mind, could cure the same symptoms if administered in homoeopathic doses.

But before this principle could be universally applied, it was necessary to make an exhaustive record of what effects various drugs would produce if administered in pure form. Dr. Hahnemann and his pupils on themselves and other healthy human beings carried out the proving. Initially, simple pills or powders were given to a number of healthy individuals whose peculiar symptoms of mind and body were noted. Thereafter, pure medicinal substances were added to these pills without telling the persons. For every drug, a record of resultant symptoms was made in detail. Simultaneously, from available medical literature, other reactions produced by the drug were noted and analyzed.

The aforesaid experiments and their results form the foundation of the homoeopathic materia medica, an exhaustive study of the effects of hundreds of drugs on the human mind and body conducted over a period of time and consisting of remarkable drug pictures.

Dr. Hahnemann made a theory, " Every effective remedy incites in the human body a kind of illness peculiar to itself, the more peculiar, the more marked and the more acute, and accordingly the medicine is the more effective." He found that every drug produced unique effects and that no two drugs were alike. This uniqueness related to production of symptoms and not to treatment of diseases. He ruled that this uniqueness was to be used for achieving a cure, to restore health to the sick by concentrating on characteristic symptoms manifested in a sick state, symptoms, which could be identified as unique and reliable to a drug.

But there was a snag. Drugs in pure administration produced an adverse reaction resulting in symptoms of sickness.

Dr. Hahnemann with a firm faith in his doctrine of *'Similia Similibus Curentur'*, started administering potencized, pure substances reduced through a special process of dilution to a negligible physical quantity in the dose which was administered to a sick person. After repeated trials, he came to the conclusion that to obtain a cure and to avoid adverse reactions, the administration of medicine in pure form could be done away with most of the time. Dr. Hahnemann found that the potencized drug had a tremendous power to cure the symptoms, which the same drug in pure form would have produced in a healthy person. He had arrived at the Everest of Medical Science.

In the orthodox practice of homoeopathy it has been the belief that only one remedy should be given at a time. There is no doubt there is drug interaction in multiple prescriptions, but it has been necessary at times when the apparent symptoms are not covered by one medicine, to administer two different medicines, either alternately or in succession. No adverse reaction has been noticed except in certain cases where the drugs are inimical to each other.

Quite contrary to the belief held by some, homoeopathy is a scientific system. Following well-laid procedures has developed the principles of homoeopathy. The proof of the pudding lies in eating. 'Like cures like' has been applied as a principle to more than a thousand drugs and to millions of patients. The results have been excellent each time. 'Proving a medicine by administering a pure substance to a healthy person is a scientific method, as scientific as there ever was. It has to be remembered that' proving' is not done to achieve a cure, but only to formulate a basis for what can be cured by a particular drug. It is but a stage in the process of research. What is seen, what is experienced, what is felt, is recorded and what the record shows simultaneously in hundreds of cases, is made the basis for coming to the conclusion that a certain drug produces certain symptoms. By no stretch of imagination can this be called unscientific. Simultaneously, the preparation of potencized medicine also follows a definite system and there is no guesswork involved at any stage. The results achieved in myriads of prescriptions of potencized medicine provide the solid rock of scientific proof on which homoeopathy stands and shines. Homoeopathy is like pure gold, which does not require a certificate to prove its value. It has stood the test of time & usage.

No reasonable person or government can overlook the benefits of the homoeopathic system of medicine. Firstly, as pointed out above, homoeopathic medicines are non-toxic. They do not have any side effects. Secondly, very few visits to the doctor are required. It is possible for literate people to take care of their day-to-day problems through a study of available homoeopathic literature. Thirdly, it is not necessary to go to a pathological laboratory unless one faces a serious problem. The homoeopathic treatment is symptomatic treatment. Symptoms as apparent are recorded and analyzed in order to choose a medicine. Fourthly, the cost of medicine is negligible. It is not a burden even on the poorest of the poor.

As has so often happened in the history of scientific progress, an accident gave Dr. Hahnemann a new insight into the effects of overdosing. " A Case of Rapidly Cured Colicodymia", which he published in 1797, tells of a patient who believed he had a tapeworm in his digestive system. He had already tried more than sixteen allopathic remedies without success. Dr. Hahnemann, working on the principle of "Like cure Like", prescribed for him Veratrum Alb.

The patient was given 4 powders of 4 grains to be taken in single early - morning doses for four days. But the patient tried to speed up his cure and finished the medicine in less than two days. This greatly aggravated the illness and soon he was on the verge of death.

Medication was immediately stopped, and fortunately the patient recovered. The illness never recurred. Dr. Hahnemann concluded that doses were too strong and too frequent caused artificially, in an acute form, the very illness they were supposed to cure. So it was necessary to reduce the quantity of medicine in each dose.

In addition to his practice and some other jobs he had to take up, Dr. Hahnemann had been for sometime now working on the revolutionary principles that would form the basis of "The Organon", his soon to be published masterwork. But with only crude diagnostic aids available in those days, he was unable to study the internal bodily changes that caused diseases.

In " Therapy of Experience", he stated: " The curative art is a science of experience. It is occupied with the annihilation of disease by helpful remedies. The knowledge of the diseases, the knowledge of the helpful remedies and the knowledge of their application form the art of healing. Even though we may not able to discover the internal bodily changes underlying the diseases, yet a survey of their external causes is of some avail. No change takes place without cause. Diseases must have their causes of origin, however much they remain hidden from us in most cases.

The internal nature of every disease, of every individual case of disease, is expressed by the existing symptoms, as far as it behaves us to know for purposes of curing"

Here we see the development of his theory that the outward symptoms are manifestations of the internal disease, and so are crucial to diagnosis and the prescription of medicine. He was sure at this stage that the smallness of a dose did not matter. If the medicine were correct, it would definitely help the body fight the disease. In fact he believed large doses aggravated the disease, because any medicinal substance could cause an adverse reaction unless administered in a proper dose.

At this stage, this great chemist turned his attention to the nature of poisons. " Medicines become poisonous simply by imperfect use; in themselves no medicines are poisonous. Ignorance frequently causes death by an overdose of medicine wrongly applied, even though the medicine may be weak enough. On the other hand, the true physician frequently saves the patients suffering from the most dangerous and peculiar symptoms, by careful use of the strongest medicines".

He was already thinking in terms of using the tenth of medicine or, for the stronger medicines, the hundredth or the thousandth or even, for the very strongest, the trillionth and quintillionth. He could see no reason why the more potent drugs, used in very small doses, should be dismissed as poison. According to him the greater the effect of a dose on the healthy human organism, the greater its medicinal value. He dared his contemporaries to free themselves from their preconceptions and think for themselves.

In the proving of medicines Dr. Hahnemann again broke new ground. In investigating the effect of medicinal potencies on healthy subjects homoeopathy reached its pinnacle. For the first time, the exact action of a drug on the human body could be scientifically studied and proved. Guesswork was eliminated.

His growing practice and teaching engagements in Leipsic left him very little time. Even so between 1181 and 1821 he managed to complete, in 6 parts, "Materia Medica Pura". But working conditions in Leipsic had become intolerable. He was friendless in the university, except for a few devoted students. Virtually none of his professional colleagues or fellow-chemists associated with him. Finally, in June 1821, he left Leipsic to settle in Kothen, a small town with a population of 6,000.

Here, too, vested interests opposed him. But Dr. Hahnemann was nothing if not a fighter. In 1822 one of his disciples, Dr. Stapf, began the 'Archive for the Homoeopathy science of Healing' - The first periodical of homoeopathy. In it, replies to various challenges posed to Dr. Hahnemann were published. In 1825 essays began appearing on the great man's life and works.

In 1828 was published 'Chronic Diseases', His last great work. Since 1816, he had been working on the resistance of many serious sicknesses to homoeopathic medicines. The treatment of chronic illnesses has exercised the minds of physicians for centuries, and even today there are no satisfactory answers.

On 10th August 1829, Dr. Hahnemann's disciples and friends celebrated the golden jubilee of his doctorate. On 31st March 1830, his wife died. She had borne him 11 children. Here was a man of 76 thinking clearly and coming up with wide-ranging solutions to a disease that used to cause widespread havoc. The concluding chapter of Dr. Hahnemann's life begins almost like a novel. By now he was settled in Kothen. On 8th October 1834, Mademoiselle Marie Melanie D'Hervilly entered his life as a patient. On 18th January 1835, they married.

In April 1843, at the age of 88, he fell ill. His condition gradually deteriorated. At 5 a.m. on 2nd July 1843 at his home in No. 1, Rue de Milan, he passed away.

The manner of his burial was shocking and inexplicable, especially for so remarkable a man. On 11th July his wife had him buried in Montmartre cemetery-without priest, prayer, or funeral music. The time of the burial was kept a secret, and nobody was invited.

So ended the life of a giant. He founded a system of medicine that was to benefit generations. He personally proved 100 medicines, "wrote more than 70 original works on chemistry and medicine, running into several thick volumes and translated about 24 works from English, French, Italian and Latin on chemistry, agriculture, and general literature". He taught, lectured, wrote hundreds of letters. In addition to his extensive practice he took an interest in subjects as diverse as Botany, Astronomy, Meteorology and Geography. An accomplished writer, he used German with wit, vigor and sensitivity. He mastered many languages.

Today, homoeopathy is practiced in many countries. Those who have benefited from the system thinks of Dr. Samuel Hahnemann with gratitude and affection. Their number grows everyday- and with it, the reputation of that great man.

CHAPTER 2

Homoeopathic System of Healing

Dr. Samuel Hahnemann laid down the fundamentals of the then new doctrine of homoeopathy in organon of medicine. As observed by him in the 'Introduction' to this work, till then no one had ever taught this homoeopathic mode of cure, no one had carried it out in practice.

Dr. Hahnemann was of the view that the art of the medical practice "should. Rapidly and mildly, effect an unalloyed and permanent cure, and restore to health by means of the smallest doses of a few simple medicines carefully selected according to their proved effect, by the only therapeutic law comfortable to nature, that is Similia Similibus Curentur".

Homoeopathy is based on the following principles:

"The physicians high and only mission is to restore the sick to health, to cure, as it is termed"

The highest ideal of cure is rapid, gentle and permanent restoration of health or removal and annihilation of the disease in its whole extent in the shortest, most reliable and most harmless way on easily comprehensible principles.

Unprejudiced observer of a sick person takes note of nothing in every individual's disease except the changes in the health of the body and of the mind, which can be perceived externally by means of the senses. "All these perceptible signs represent the disease in its whole extent, that is, together they form the true and only conceivable portrait of the disease"

"A single one of the symptoms present is no more the disease itself than a single foot is the man himself"

As far as the doctor is concerned, the disease merely consists of the totality of its symptoms. He needs only to eradicate these in order to cure the disease. The cause, which gives rise to the illness or perpetuates it, is to be removed. A palliative treatment centered round one single symptom should not be considered.

"As this natural law of cure manifests itself in every pure experiment, it matters little what may be the scientific explanation of how it takes place".

"Every real medicine at all times under all circumstances, on every living human being, and produced in time its peculiar symptoms, distinctly perceptible, if the dose be large enough".

"In order that a medicine may effect a cure, it is before all things requisite that it should be capable of producing in the human body an artificial disease as similar as possible to the disease to be cured".

Even the uncommonly small doses of medicine used in the homoeopathic cure, after destruction of the malady, leave a certain trace of medicinal disease in the organism. But, on account of extraordinary minuteness of the dose, this trace is so transient, so slight that it disappears rapidly of its own accord.

A natural disease can never be cured by medicines that posses the power of producing in the healthy individual an alien, morbid state, and symptoms which differ from those of the disease to be cured.

The only possible mode of treatment of disease is the homoeopathic one in which there is employed for the totality of the symptoms of a natural disease, a medicine capable of producing the most similar symptoms possible in the healthy individual, given in a suitable dose.

The first part of a physician's job is to know the totality of the symptoms of a sick person. The second part of this knowledge is to know as to what affects a medicine in it pure form can produce on a healthy individual. This power of medicine can only be observed by administering them in gross doses to healthy human beings. If in order to ascertain the effect of a medicine on a human system it is given to a sick person, little or nothing precise can be seen of its true effects because the peculiar alterations of the health to be expected from the medicine are mixed up with the symptoms of the disease and can be seldom be distinctively observed.

" Therefore medicines, on which depend mans life and death, disease and health, must be thoroughly and most carefully distinguished from one another, and for this purpose tested by this careful, pure experiments on the healthy body for the purpose of ascertaining there powers and real effects, in order to obtain an accurate knowledge of them, and to enable us to avoid any mistake in their employment in diseases, for it is only by correct selection of them that the greatest of all earthly blessings, the health of the body and of the mind can be rapidly and permanently restored".

For proving a medicine it must be taken in a perfectly simple, unadulterated form. It must be employed quiet alone, without the admixture of any foreign substance and without taking anything else of a medicinal nature the same day. Throughout the experiment the diet of the person on whom the experiment is being conducted must be strictly regulated. The person who is proving the medicine must be preeminently trustworthy and conscientious and during the experiment, he should avoid all overexertion and disturbing passions. He must devote himself to careful self-observation and must not be disturbed whilst so engaged. The medicines must be tested on both males and females, in order to reveal the alterations of the health they produce in the sexual sphere.

The more moderate the doses of the medicine used for such experiments are, so much the more distinctly are the primary effects developed, and only these are most worth knowing.

All the sufferings, accidents and changes of the health of the experimenter during the action of the medicines are solely derived from the medicine and must be regarded and registered as belonging peculiarly to this medicine. The symptoms in such an experiment do not arise spontaneously but are produced by the medicine.

"If we have thus tested on the healthy individual a considerable number of simple medicines and carefully and faithfully registered all the disease elements and symptoms they are capable of developing as artificial disease producers, then only have we a true materia medica- a collection is real, pure, reliable modes of action of simple medicinal substances, a volume of the book of nature, where in is recorded a considerable array of the peculiar changes of the health and symptoms ascertained to belong to each of the powerful medicines.

"The third point of the business of a true physician relates to the judicious employment of the artificial morbific agents (medicines) that have been proved on healthy individuals to ascertain their pure action, in order to effect the homoeopathic cure of natural disease".

"Among the lists of symptoms of many medicines it will not be difficult to find one from whose separate disease elements a type of curative artificial disease, very like the totality of the symptoms of the natural disease, may be constructed, such a medicine is the desired remedy."

" In this search for a homoeopathic specific remedy, that is to say, in this comparison of the collective symptoms of the natural disease with the list of symptoms of known medicines, in order to find among these an artificial morbific agent corresponding by similarity to the disease to be cured, the more striking, singular, uncommon and peculiar (characteristic) signs and symptoms of the selected medicine must correspond to, in order to constitute it the most suitable for effecting the cure. The most general and undefined symptoms: The more general and undefined symptoms, loss of appetite, headache, debility, restless sleep, discomfort, and so forth, demand but little attention when of that vague and indefinite character, if they cannot be more accurately described, as symptoms of such a general nature are observed in almost every disease and from almost every drug".

"If the antitype constructed from the list of symptoms of the most suitable medicine contain those peculiar, uncommon, singular and distinguishing (characteristic) symptoms, which are to be met with in the disease to be cured in the greatest number and in the greatest similarity, this medicine is the most appropriate homoeopathic specific remedy for this morbid state; the disease, if it be not one of very long standing, will generally be removed and extinguished by the first dose of it, without any considerable disturbance."

A homoeopathic dose may cause a kind of slight aggravation when the dose has not been sufficiently small or has been somewhat too large for a few hours. This aggravation has a resemblance to the original disease. In reality it is nothing more than an extremely similar medicinal disease, somewhat exceeding in strength the original affection. This slight homoeopathic aggravation during the first hours is a very good prognostic that the acute disease will most probably yield to the first dose.

In chronic cases, such increase of the original symptoms can appear only at the end of the treatment when the cure is almost or quite finished.

The external treatment of a disease having purely local symptoms is always injurious. The source of such a disease lies in some internal malady. No external malady can arise, persist or even grow worse without some internal cause. No eruption on the lips, no whitlow can occur without previous or simultaneous ill health. "All true medical treatment of a disease on the external parts of the body that has occurred from little or no injury from without must, therefore, be directed against the whole, must effect the annihilation and cure of the general malady by means of internal remedies, if it is wished that the treatment should be judicious, sure, efficacious and radical."

All chronic ills and maladies must be healed from the inside by homoeopathic means, after information of previous treatment has been obtained.

The so-called diseases of the mind and temperament, intermittent diseases and intermittent fever can be treated by homoeopathy.

"In all cases of disease we are called on to cure, the state of the patients disposition is to be particularly noted, along with the totality of the symptoms, if we could trace an accurate picture of the disease, in order to be able thereof to treat it homoeopathically with success."

In chronic cases a carefully selected medicine may be given daily and for months, if necessary. A start may be made with a low degree of potency for a few weeks. Thereafter, a change may be made to a higher degree.

"A fundamental principle of the homoeopathic physician (which distinguishes him from every physician of all older schools) is this, that he never employs for any patient a medicine, whose effect on the healthy human has not previously been carefully proven and thus made known to him."

□□□

CHAPTER 3

Hahnemann Tips on Examining A Patient

This individualizing examination of a case of disease, for which Dr. Hahnemann give general directions, of which the practitioner will bear in mind only what is applicable for each individual case, demands of the physician nothing but freedom from prejudice and sound senses, attention in observing and fidelity in tracing the picture of the disease.

The patient details the history of his sufferings; those about him tell what they heard him complain of, how he has behaved and what they have noticed in him; the physician sees, hears, and remarks by his other senses what there is of an altered or unusual character about him. He writes down accurately all that the patient and his friends have told him in the very expressions used by them. Keeping silence himself, he allows them to say all they have to say, and refrains from interrupting them (every interruption breaks the train of thought of the narrators, and all they would have said at first does not again occur to them in precisely the same manner after that.) unless they wander off to other matters. The physician advises them at the beginning of the examination to speak slowly, in order that he may take down in writing the important parts of what the speaker says.

He begins a fresh line with every new circumstance mentioned by the patient or his friends, so that the symptoms shall be all ranged separately one below the other. He can thus add to any one that may at first have been related in too vague a manner but subsequently more explicitly explained.

When the narrator have finished what they would say of their own accord, the physician than reverts to each particular symptom and elicits more precise information respecting to in the following manner; he reads over the symptoms as they were related to him one by one, amid about each of them he inquires for further particulars e.g. at what period did the symptoms occurs? Was it previous to taking the medicine he had hitherto been using? Whilst taking the medicine? Or only some days after leaving off the medicine? What kind of pain, what sensation exactly, was it that occurred on this spot? Did the pain occur in fits and by itself, at various times? Or was it continued, without intermission? How long did it last? And what time of the day/night, and in what position of the body was it worst, or ceased entirely? What was the exact nature of this or that event or circumstance mentioned - described in plain words?

And thus the physician obtains more precise information respecting each particular detail, but without ever framing his questions so as to suggest the answer to the patient, (for instance the physician should not ask, was not this or that circumstance present? He should never be guilty of making such suggestions, which tend to seduce the patient into giving a false answer and a false account of his symptoms) so that he shall only have to answer yes or no; else he will be misled to answer in the affirmative or negative something untrue, half true, or not strictly correct, wither from indolence or in order to please his interrogator, from which a false picture of the disease and an unsuitable mode of treatment must result.

If in these voluntary details nothing has been mentioned respecting several; facts or functions of the body or his mental state, the physician asks what more can be told in regard to these parts and these functions, or the state of his disposition or mind: (for example what is the character of his stools? How does he pass his water? How is it with his day and night sleep? What is the state of his disposition, his humour, and his memory? How about the thirst? What sort of taste has he in his mouth? What kind of foods and drink are most relished? What are most repugnant to him? Has each its full natured taste, or some other unusual taste? How does he feel after eating or drinking? Has he anything to tell about the head, the limbs or the abdomen?) But in doing this he only makes use of general expressions, in order that his informants may be obliged to enter onto special details concerning them.

When the patient (for it is on him we have chiefly to rely for a description of his sensations, except in the case of feigned disease) has by these details, given of his own accord and in answer to inquiries, furnished the requisite information and traced a tolerably perfect picture of the disease, the physician is at liberty and obliged (if he feels he has not yet gained all the information he needs) to ask more precise, more special questions. (For example how often his bowels are moved? What is the exact character of the stools? Did the whitish evacuation consist of mucus or faeces? Had he or had he not pains during the evacuations? What was their exact character, and where were they seated? What did the patient vomit? Is the bad taste in the mouth putrid, or bitter, or sour, or what? Before or after eating? At what period of the day was it worst? What is the taste of what is eructated? Does the urine only become turbid on standing, or is it turbid on standing, or is it turbid when first discharged? What is its colour when first emitted? Of what colour is the sediment? How does he behave during sleep? Does he whine? Moan, talk or cry out in his sleep?

Does he start during sleep? Does he snore during inspiration, or during expiration? Does he lie only on his back, or on which side? Does he cover himself well up, or can he not bear the clothes on him? Does he easily awake, or does sleep too soundly? How does he feel immediately after waking from sleep? How often does this or that symptom occur? What is the cause that produces it each time it occurs? Does it come on whilst sitting, lying standing, or when in motions? Only when fasting, or in the morning, or only in the evening, or only after a meal, or when does it usually appear? When did the rigor come on? Was it merely a chilly sensation, or was he actually cold at the same time? If so, in what parts? Or while feeling chilly, was he actually warm to the touch? Was it merely a sensation of cold, without shivering? Was he hot without redness of the face? What parts of him were hot to the touch? Or did he complain of heat without being hot to the touch? How long did the chilliness last? How long the hot stage? When did the thirst come on- during the cold stage? During the heat or previous to it or subsequently to it? How great was the thirst, and what was the beverage desired? When did the sweat come on- at the beginning or at the end of the heat? Or how many hours after the heat? When asleep or when awake? How great was the sweat? Was it warm or cold? On what parts? How did it smell? What does he complain of before or during the cold stage/ what during the hot stage? What after it? What during or after the sweating stage?

In women, note the character of menstruation and other discharges, etc)

When the physician has finished writing down these particulars, he then makes a note of what he himself observes in the patient,) for example, how the patient behaved during the visit- whether he was morose, quarellersome, hasty, lachrymose, anxious, despairing or safe or hopeful, calm etc. whether he was in a drowsy state or in any way dull of comprehension; whether he spoke hoarsely, or in a low tone, or in coherently, or how otherwise did he talk? What was the color of his face and eyes, and of his skin generally? What degree of liveliness and power was there in his expression and eyes? What was the state of his tongue, his breathing, the smell from his mouth, and his hearing? Were his pupils dilated or contracted? How rapidly and to what extent did they alter in the dark and in the light? What was the character of the pulse? What the condition of the abdomen? How moist or hot, how cold or dry to the touch, was the skin of this or that part or generally? Whether he lay with head thrown back, with mouth half or wholly open, with the arms placed above the head, on his back, or in what other position? What effort did he make to raise himself? And anything else in him that may strike the physician as being remarkable) and ascertains how much of that was peculiar to the patient in his healthy state.

In chronic diseases of females, it is especially necessary to pay attention to pregnancy, sterility, sexual desire, miscarriages and the state of the menstrual discharge. With respect to the last named more particularly, we should not neglect to ascertain if it recurs at too short intervals, or is delayed beyond the proper time, how many days it lasts, whether its flow is continuous or interrupted, what is its general quantity, how dark is its colour, whether there is leucorrhoea before its appearance or after its termination, but especially by what bodily or mental ailments, what sensations and pains, it is preceded, accompanied or followed; if there is leucorrhoea, what is its nature, what sensation attend its flow, in what quantity it is, and what are the conditions and occasions under which it occurs.

By and large, the use of one properly selected medicine should bring about amelioration. The patient would experience " a greater degree of comfort, increased calmness and freedom of mind, higher spirits- a kind of return of the natural state."

CHAPTER 4

Selection of Remedy

Homoeopathic treatment is based on an overall understanding of the symptoms in the body and mind created by a sickness. Dr. Samuel Hahnemann, the founder of the homoeopathic science of healing, after years of experiment and trial, came to finding that symptom - similarity is the curative method of medically curable diseases. In paragraph 25 of the 'Organon of Medicine', he formulated the principle of 'like cures like' in these words: " Now, however, in all careful trials, pure experience, the sole and infallible oracle of the healing art, teaches us that actually that medicine which, in its action on the healthy human body, has demonstrated its power of producing the greatest number of symptoms similar to those observable in the case of disease under treatment, does also, rapidly, radically and permanently remove the totality of the symptoms of this morbid state, that is to say, the whole disease present, and change it into health; and that all medicines cure, without exception, those diseases whose symptoms most really resemble their own, and leave none of them uncured."

The aforesaid indicates the importance of symptoms in the diagnosis and treatment in homoeopathy. If a drug creates a symptom during the course of proving, then it can be cured by a potencised dose of the drug; whatever may be the name of the disease. For instance, in proving GLONOINE produces a bursting, throbbing sensation in the head in a healthy person. Conversely any surging of the blood to the head requires GLONOINE. This can happen in a sun - stroke, in high blood pressure, in cerebro - spinal meningitis. KALI BICROMICUM produces in proving, a tough, stringy discharge of mucus. In homoeopathy, KALI BICROMICUM cures a similar discharge whether from the nose inwards from mouth, from fauces, from pharynx, from larynx, trachea, bronchi, vagina, and uterus or from any mucus membrane. CACTUSGRANDIFLORUS produces in pure form and gross doses, constriction of the heat and a constriction, anywhere in the body, which is like an iron band being tightened. The same sensation of constriction leads us to the use of CACTUS in a homoeopathic dose and it need not be confined to the heart. There can be constriction of the scalp, in the oesophagus, in the chest, in the abdomen, bladder, uterus, vagina or rectum.

The human body is a very sensitive instrument and when there is suffering, its sensibility is heightened.

Ask the patient to tell you about his state of mind and to describe in his own words what is being experienced by him while suffering from a particular sickness. Besides, observe what is apparent and note it on a paper carefully. Slight differences in symptoms can lead to a different prescription. To illustrate, in a day-to-day problem like common cold, the discharge of mucus can be of different types. The thickness, the flow, the colour of the discharge help in deciding upon the choice of the medicine. Extremely acrid, copious discharge, nose dripping like a tap, along-with eyes watering profusely may indicate the need for ALLUM CEPA. On the other hand, the same excoriating, thin and copious discharge may require ARSENIC ALB if there is burning and restlessness. At other times, the discharge may be full of pus, blood and may have a stinking smell. There is pain deep in the nose. The chosen medicine may be AURUM MET. Another discharge in cold can be thick, ropy, greenish, flowing inwards into the mouth and very difficult to take out. This is accompanied by pain in the sinuses. Here, we shall choose KALI BICHROMICUM. But, if the discharge is green, bland, comes outwards, is abundant in the morning, the medicine would be PULSATILLA.

It would be noticed how a slight variation in the symptoms has led to the selection of a different remedy. This is so because every drug produces peculiar changes in the human mind and body and such changes are not produced in the same manner by any other medicinal substance. There can be, from a medical point of view, no equivalent remedies whatsoever, no surrogates., (Organon, Footnote 79). To illustrate, let us take tonsillitis-the tonsils are swollen inflamed, red, painful, shining and dry. The patient generally has fever. BELLADONNA is required.

But if the colour of the tonsils is purple, although there is pain and inflammation, the drug required is LACHESIS. Further, the tonsils may have pus, which can be seen in the shape of white patches on the surface of the tonsils and of the throat. This pus at times can be painful and sometimes not. There is difficulty in swallowing. We choose HEPAR SULPH when there is a shooting, piercing, stabbing and throbbing pain on swallowing or otherwise and when pus has been formed. But if in spite of formation of pus, the degree of shooting pain were less, MERC SOL would give instant relief. On the other hand, if the stabbing pain on swallowing is there, but pus is not visible BARYTA CARB would be the correct medicine.

The mental state of the patient plays a great part in the selection of homoeopathic remedies. In the experiments conducted with drugs to discover their effect on healthy human beings, a careful note was taken of changes produced in the mental state of the person. Hundreds of thousands of such variations were noted and analyzed. In turn, these very variations as exhibited by the sick person help in the identification of the drug, which is his remedy. For instance, restlessness of mind and body, tossing about, anxiety, nervousness and fear, irrational or otherwise, would indicate the need for ACONITE. On the other hand, fear of apprehension, failure in the examination, fear of one's own insufficiency, may indicate the need for ARGENTUM NITRICUM. Its proving also include confusion in thinking, depression, melancholy and a slowing down of mental activity.

Everyone is aware that the course of sickness is cut short by certain changes in the physical environment. Similarly, sickness can be aggravated by other changes in climate, because of change in diet, on account of physical movement and so on. Hence, it is necessary while examining the patient to find out if there is any circumstance on the happening of which his sickness is ameliorated or aggravated. To illustrate: discharge from an ear is quite a common problem. This discharge has certain colour. A certain type of pain also accompanies it. A mucous discharge with blood, pulsating pain and throbbing in the ear, if better when the patient is lying on the painful side, in dry weather, requires CALCAREA CARB. This discharge would be worse in cold weather or on exposure to air. On the other hand, if the discharge is foul smelling, is accompanied by throbbing in the ear, but is less in wrapping in the head up, or with warmth or is worse from dry cold wind or when the patient is lying on the painful side, it requires HEPAR SULPH. Please notice the distinction. The CALC CARB patient is better lying on the painful side. The HEPAR SULPH patient is worse lying on the painful side.

Take another common problem. Pain in muscles. Shooting pain in limbs, which might come on exposure to dry cold air, would require ACONITE. There is numbness and tingling. Pain comes on suddenly and violently. The patient is fearful and anguished. Another muscular pain may come on account of an injury. The medicine indicated is ARNICA. On the other hand, pain in muscles, increasing in severity gradually with joints inflamed and red hot, needs BRYONIA. This pain is better from firm and strong pressure but is worse on movement. Muscular pain, which is temporarily ameliorated on movement or from change of position, needs RHUS TOX. Between BRYONIA and RHUS TOX, one of the distinguishing symptoms is aggravation on movement in the case of BRYONIA and a temporary relief on movement in the case of RHUS TOX. There are other differentiating symptoms too which ought to be taken into account. But, even if the aforesaid one distinction were kept in mind, the choice of the medicine would not be wrong.

It is these, which differentiate one drug from another. The mental and nervous symptoms rank very high in the selection of remedies. General symptoms have an important place but local exceptions cannot be overlooked. Common symptoms, which every patient has, are of less value. However, apparently unimportant or trivial symptoms such as the reaction of the patient to his environment must not be ignored because we are creatures of our environment. A person suffering from chronic rheumatic arthritis with paralytic affections and progressive loss of muscular strength may be restless at night. While he is better by heat or warm application, in damp and wet weather, he is worse in dry weather. He requires CAUSTICUM. Another patient suffering from a similar malady is better in dry weather, is also better by warmth. But, he cannot tolerate cold fresh air. His joints are hot, swollen and painful. He is depressed, is weary of life, and is mentally confused. He is restless and full of anxiety. He requires RHUS TOX. Thus, minute distinctions in the visible mental and physical symptoms or in the modalities of symptoms, that is to say, amelioration or aggravation, occurring in certain circumstances, help us in the selection of proper homoeopathic medicines.

Sensation plays a great part in the identification of sickness in any medical system, but more so in homoeopathy. Quite often, we select a medicine on the basis of sensations. With experience, diagnosis becomes easy. It may be worthwhile to go through the few pages devoted to a particular symptoms or problem to the end before deciding upon a medicine for a particular diseased condition. Normally, this would take only a few minutes. For instance, the colour of the stool is an important indication in the treatment of loose motions. The colour of the stool varies according to the different causes for the upset.

There are problems like dysentery, which have troubled mankind for thousand of years. Every system of medicine has tried to find a long-term cure for this disorder of the intestines. It is only homoeopathy, which has found medicine, which not only takes care of dysentery but also at the same time, do not destroy the healthy bacteria in the digestive system. To obtain this advantage, if you have to go through symptoms of eight different medicines, the effort is worthwhile because the exercise would not have to be repeated and the patient would get lasting relief.

For acute problems, repeat medicines in a low potency such as 30, if necessary, every 15 or 30 minutes till the condition of the patient stabilizes. Thereafter, the potency can be raised as indicated and the number of doses reduced to four per day, should be limited to four in 24 hours. Wherever the frequency of the dose is less, it has been indicated.

In chronic cases the correctly selected medicines has to be administered in a high potency such as 200, 1000 or above, four times a day for quite a few days, even weeks. Recovery sets in slowly, imperceptibly till a cure occurs. If a stage comes when recovery stops midway, it is time to increase the potency.

By and large, the use of one properly selected medicine should bring about amelioration. The patient would experience "a greater degree of comfort, increased calmness and freedom of mind, high spirits - a kind of return of the natural state."

Absence of amelioration indicates choice of a wrong remedy. If the symptoms are so varied that one medicine does not cover them, more than one medicine may be taken but the medicine should not be mixed and should be taken at an interval of 30 minutes or more. Medicines, which are inimical to each other, should not be taken in succession. Drug administration should be stopped as soon as recovery occurs. There is no fixed duration for which drugs are to be taken. Use of drugs beyond the stage of recovery brings the disease back. An aggravation occurs. As you stop the medicine, the aggravation disappears.

❑❑❑

CHAPTER 5

Homoeopathic Materia Medica

The homoeopathic materia medica consists of around 1000 drugs, the characteristics of which have been verified or proved. Homoeopathy is unique in that it uses no drug, which has not been proved. The proving has been done by administering pure medicines to healthy human beings and recording in minute detail the effects, mostly adverse, produced by such administration. The tests were conducted on men and women who were mostly medical people and students who were not sick. The drugs were administered in doses consisting of crude drugs or homoeopathic potencies. These volunteers were then asked to describe the effects of the drugs in their own words. These descriptions were noted down by the doctors conducting the experiments and were carefully recorded. Hundreds of thousands of such symptoms were recorded while proving the homoeopathic drugs and the materia medica forms a record of the best proving along with other data collected as a result of laboratory tests and experiments.

In paragraph 25 of the 'Organon of medicine', Dr.Samuel Hahnemann the founder of the system laid down the basis of homoeopathy in the following words: "Now, however, in all careful trials, pure experience, the sole and infallible oracle of healing art, teaches us that medicine which, in its action on the healthy human body, has demonstrated its power of producing the greatest number of symptoms similar to those observable in the case of disease under treatment, does also, in doses of suitable potency and attenuation, rapidly, radically and permanently remove the totality of the symptoms of this morbid state, that is to say the whole disease present, and change it into health; and that all medicines cure, without exception, those diseases whose symptoms most nearly resemble their own, and leave none of them uncured."

The limitations of drugs used in other systems of medicine have been known all along. Even today, despite the considerable progress made in medical science, doctors and pharmacologists depend a good deal on the body to cure itself. No class of drugs, except those that cure infections, can really treat the basic causes or the underlying processes of diseases. They can relieve pain or discomfort; they can limit and prevent the consequences of some diseases; sometimes they even counteract diseases to the extent of establishing near normalcy in the body.

To find a way out of the difficulties that were being experienced (and that are being experienced even today) regarding the knowledge of the effects of particular drugs on human beings, Dr. Hahnemann started the proving of medicines on healthy persons. This was the rock on which the foundation of homoeopathic materia medica rested. In paragraph 143 of the Organon of Medicine, Dr. Hahnemann came to the conclusion that, "if we have tested on the healthy individual a considerable number of simple medicines and carefully and faithfully registered all the disease elements and symptoms they are capable of developing as artificial disease producers, then only we have a true materia medica- a collection of real, pure, reliable modes of action of simple medicinal substances, a volume of the book of nature, wherein is recorded a considerable array of the peculiar changes of the health and symptoms ascertained to belong to each of the powerful medicines, as they were revealed to the attention of the observer, in which the likeness of the (homoeopathic) disease elements of many natural diseases to be hereafter cured by them are present, which, in a word, contain artificial morbid states, that furnish for the similar natural morbid states the only true, homoeopathic that is to say, specific, therapeutics instruments for effecting their certain and permanent cure.

It is a matter of considerable significance that the effects of the drugs in their pure form were studied in human beings and not animals because human beings can describe what happens to them after a drug has been administered while an animal's responses can only be seen or measured or tested in a laboratory. A rat cannot tell us that it has pain in the stomach and that a particular drug has lessened the severity of pain. Similarly the effect of a drug on the mind of an animal cannot really be known except by watching its behavioural aberrations. No such limitation binds a human being. Therein lies the superiority of the homoeopathic materia medica.

It is common knowledge today that quite a few drugs used in the allopathic pharmacopoeia while helping one function of the body, interfere with another. A very large number of drugs have for this reason to be continuously balanced. Prescriptions of antibiotics are accompanied by prescriptions of multivitamins preparations. Corticosteriods used to dilate the bronchial tubes in asthma are prescribed without understanding their action. A prolonged use of these medicines adversely affected the health of the patient and he develops hoarseness and thrush in the mouth. Most drugs prescribed to reduce blood pressure have powerful aide effects and the doctors are always struggling to balance the risk in taking these drugs with the risk of raised blood pressure itself.

The homoeopathic materia medica on the other hand, long ago, almost totally reversed the possibility of adverse effects of drugs by potencization, that is by reducing the quantity of drug used for a cure to levels, which cannot be tested even in a laboratory. Potencization served more than one purpose. It reduced the adverse effects of a drug and brought out its inherent healing powers in direct proportion to its dilution.

A study of the materia medica thus provides the reader a glimpse into an extremely fascinating part of the spectrum of homoeopathy. As stated above, the homoeopathic *materia* medica is the result of a very scientific study of the effects of drugs on healthy human beings. Dr. Burnett, an eminent author, called homoeopathy 'Scientific Medicine'. Dr. M.L. Tyler, a writer on the *materia* medica, described it as 'medicine based on ascertained facts and abundantly proved deductions'. According to him, the wider our knowledge and the more conscientiously applied, the better results we get. He went on to say, "But, while considering the cure of curable sickness by the Therapy of Likes, there are incurable cases of diseases, or results of diseases. You cannot put back lung tissue that has ulcerated out, any more than you can readjust an amputated limb, so that it shall survive and function normally. But, for the most incurable cases the Medicine of Likes still holds good. It may and does palliate and indefinitely prolong life. What is left of the ulcerated lung may heal and suffice to carry on with -even for years. Besides which, who shall dogmatize as to what is incurable? Homoeopathy in the hands of courageous, enthusiastic and imaginative physicians, can narrow down the range of incurability: can even work seeming miracles of healing."

Such seeming miracles of healing are being worked by the use of homoeopathic medicines every day in millions of cases. No better proof of this can be seen than in the action of Sulphur which Dr. E.B. Nash as American authority on the homoeopathic material medica has called one of the monuments to the genius of Hahnemann.

According to the homoeopathic materia medica, Veratrum Alb is the medicine in cholera, in stool, which is copious, of rice colour, uncontrollable and which is accompanied by non-stop retching. The patient has cold sweat on the face and a cold and blue skin. Administration of one dose of Veratrum Alb 1000 improves such a patient to an extent that his retching is controlled immediately and so is his diarrhoea. He goes to sleep in short whole and wakes up cured.

A thorough study of the materia medica is of great help in the choice of the best homoeopathic remedy for symptoms exhibited in the mind and body of the patient. It cannot be anyone's case that all the symptoms as produced in a healthy human being in proving with a particular drug would be present at the same time in a patient Dr. Hahnemann was aware of this situation. In paragraph 153 of 'Organon of Medicine', he observed that the "more striking, singular, uncommon and peculiar (characteristic) signs and symptoms of the case of the disease are chiefly and most likely to be kept in view." These, in particular, ought to correspond with similar ones in the list of symptoms of the selected medicine. " The more general and undefined symptoms: loss of appetite, headache, debility, restless sleep, discomfort and so forth, demand but little attention" when these are of vague and indefinite character and can only be observed in almost every disease and for almost every drug.

The ' individuality of each drug is a revolutionary finding. No two drugs are alike in nature. Most drugs in their pure administration generate symptoms in the human mind and body, which are adverse to what is known as sound health. Amongst these symptoms some are very distinguishing, characteristic and stand out as unique. These symptoms act as a lighthouse for the physician in search of a drug in a particular situation. It may be necessary in a particular situation to first utilize one drug to exhaust and ameliorate most of the symptoms of the patient and then follow it up with another drug to cover the symptoms still not eliminated. It was realized even by Dr. Hahnemann that, "It is next to impossible that medicine and disease should cover one another symptomatically as exactly as two triangles with equal sides and equal angles."

CHAPTER 6

Homoeopathy A Success

Homoeopathy system of medicine is the system of healing suited to all the young, and the old, the rich and the poor, the people in the developed as well as the underdeveloped countries and for persons in any place or climate. This is not to take away from the value and utility of the other prevalent systems of medicine. The aim of every science of healing is the relief of sick. Every system is successful in its own fashion. Homoeopathy too fights sickness and does so with remarkable results. Additionally the cost of diagnosis in this system is negligible because the diagnosis is by and large symptomatic. The medicine itself is inexpensive. Notable efficacy and low costs are the strong points of homoeopathic medicine. There are no toxic effects of the drugs, no side effects. The time taken for the medicine to show improvement is not long. Homoeopathic medicines are easy to store and have a long life.

Homoeopathy has been attacked again and again on the ground that the potencised drugs cannot be tested in a laboratory. But that way a number of phenomenon is still outside the pale of conventional science. However, laboratory tests have been going in many countries and certain phenomenon not acceptable to conventional scientific beliefs have been observed.

The homoeopathic system of medicine develops for its special use, the inner medicinal powers of the crude substances by means of a process peculiar to it and which has never been tried, whereby they only all become immeasurably and penetratingly efficacious and remedial. Even those that in the crude state give no evidence of the slightest medicinal power on the human body.

This remarkable change in the qualities of natural bodies develops the latent, hidden powers, which influence the body, change the well-being. This is affected by mechanical action upon their smallest particles by means of rubbing and shaking and through the addition of an indifferent substance, dry or fluid. This process is called dynamization; potencizing and the products are dynamizations or potencies in different degrees.

Potencization is not to be confused with simple dilution, which does not develop the pure drug into a medicinal dose nor brings out its latent curative energy. The terms potencization and dynamization have a literal significance because the curative powers of a drug increases in direct proportion to successive homoeopathic dilutions.

To prepare a medicine of one potency on the centesimal scale one part of the drug is diluted with 99 parts of the diluent vehicle, an inert or non-medicinal substance, usually sugar of milk or rectified spirit. Shaking for about an hour mixes the drug. The resultant total has one potency.

Out of the above 100 parts of potency, one part is taken and mixed with another 99 parts of the diluent. After rubbing & shaking for another one hour, potency two is produced. Thus one can get the frequently used potencies of 30,200,1000,100000 and so on.

Today all these potencized drugs are made under scientifically controlled conditions in various laboratories with the help of modern machinery. The positive action of a potencized drug was found to be overpowering to such an extent that the insignificant adverse reaction with the drug was bound to produce on account of its nature was virtually obliterated through dynamization.

It may be difficult to imagine that in a dose, say of 10,000 potency there would be some medicine left. In the third potency the degree of dilution is one millionth. But continuous use of such potencies used by homoeopaths and the remarkable results obtained from the same in the cure of sick persons have established a new path in the field of medicine and took a quantum jump in the alleviation of human suffering by evolving the aforesaid method of potencisation.

The homoeopathic medicine from bee sting poison is called Apis. In potencized form, Apis cures all the symptoms, that is, oedema, dropsy, swelling with burning and stinging pain, constriction, stiffness and restlessness, what ever be the cause of these symptoms whether a bee sting or rheumatism or meningitis or a kidney problem.

That is homoeopathy for you. Prove a drug: note the symptoms it produces. Potencize the drug. Use the resultant medicine to the remedy in sick man the symptoms pure substance produces in healthy human beings.

Another poisonous insect, a black spider, when it bites, creates a carbuncle on the human skin. This pimple small in beginning continues to swell and spread. The patient has a chill. Fever sets in. a large abscess forms which is hard, it has been observed that carbuncles with similar symptoms can be cured with the use of the same poison known as Tarentula Cubensis made into a homoeopathic potencized dose.

Or, think of belladonna, black berries of the deadly nightshade, which cause poisoning in children. The victim's pupils are dilated; his skin becomes dry and bright red; his face is scarlet. The symptoms resemble those of scarlet fever. Belladonna in homoeopathic doses cures scarlet fever as well as any other sickness in which the above symptoms are present.

Homoeopathy is a system of medicine that uses natural substances. These natural substances come from the mineral, vegetable and animal kingdoms. Homoeopathic remedies are manufactured in a manner that does not render them toxic. There are no side effects.

Homoeopathy has used ordinary substances like vegetable charcoal and table salts for obtaining remarkable cures. Carbo Veg, which is homoeopathic preparation from vegetable charcoal, is one of the finest medicines for debility for acidity. Chronic or otherwise, and for cyanosis which refers to blueness of the skin in a number of emergencies and diseases. Natrum Mur, is common salt, it is a great medicine in homoeopathic doses, for anaemia, for debility, for intermittent fevers like malaria and for coryza.

Metals like gold, silver, platinum and minerals like sulphur, arsenic, antimony, have all been made to serve the mission of homoeopathy. Substances available in the herbal, mineral or animal kingdoms have been transformed by potencization in invaluable medicines for acute as well as chronic.

Substances, which are used as medicines, are medicines only in so far as they possess each its own way to alter the well being of man through its influence. The medicinal property of those material substances, which we call medicines, relates only to their properties to bring alterations in the human body.

Thus every special medicinal substance alters through a kind of infection, that well being of man in a peculiar manner its own and not in a manner peculiar to another medicine.

Every real medicine acts at all times, under all circumstances on every living human being and produces in time its peculiar symptoms, distinctly perceptible if the dose be large enough.

❑❑❑

PART – II

COMMON AILMENTS

CHAPTER 7

Accidents & Emergencies

This chapter provides a readily available means of reference for helping in life threatening emergencies, accidents and for providing first aid, where any delay caused by the lack of medication or non-availability of the doctor can have serious consequences either in terms of life or in terms of resulting serious sickness.

As soon as possible competent medical help should be availed of in emergencies and accidents. In the meanwhile the homoeopathic medicines suggested hereafter would provide relief, would halt deterioration in most cases and may save life in many instances.

Emergencies can be life threatening. One of these can be severe haemorrhage, where copious bleeding can lead to death. Obstruction of breathing for different reasons is a matter for concern. Serious accidents are life threatening because there may be unmanageable bleeding, shock and pain.

Below, a list of few medicines and other items required for first aid in emergencies has been given. This can be helpful in homes, in factories and offices.

Loss of Consciousness: Absence of Breathing

Precautions

1. Take the causality out of the zone of danger e.g. a house on fire or a road with traffic, by dragging.
2. Loosen collar, raise the chin up and clear the mouth with your fingers.
3. Give artificial respiration; failing this, begin chest compression.

Medicines

1. Five drops of CAMPHOR mother tincture on sugar every five minutes.

CAMPHOR drops on handkerchief to smell; but this would help only if breathing has started.

Accidents Involving Internal Injuries With Or Without Bleeding

Such accidents can cause an injury to the stomach, or to any other part of the body. There may be no open wounds, but internally there is a hemorrhage.

Precautions

Do not move the patient till the internal hemorrhage has been brought under control.

Medicines

1. ARNICA 1000 in case the accident has caused a mechanical injury, a physical trauma. Hemorrhage below the skin-surface of an injury is taken care of. Arnica prevents the skin turning blue or black. It relieves pain.
2. MILLEFOLIUM 200 to be repeated every half an hour till the internal bleeding has been controlled. The hemorrhage is of bright red blood. It can be from bowels, nose or from any other internal organs.
3. CHINA 200 to counteract weakness resulting from copious flows of blood for any reason. To be administered for a few days, 4 times a day. Restores strength.

Accidents Involving Superficial Injuries

Precautions

1. Remove the patient out of the danger zone, that is, where he might be physically injured by oncoming traffic or for any other reason.
2. Make sure that the patient can breathe comfortably.
3. Care should be taken not to touch the bleeding areas with any dirty linen.

Medicines

1. ARNICA 1000 is case the bleeding has been caused by injury.
2. CALENDULA mother tincture. Apply locally on the cuts and lacerations with a clean cotton swab. It cuts down pain and prevents pus

formation. After applying Calendula the wound can be dressed with a light bandage, if necessary.

Asphyxiation

Lack of oxygen in the blood supply can lead to death. A blocking of the mouth and nose, by physical obstruction or by a piece of bone, or by food or liquid stuck in the throat and the oesophagus can cause this. Diseases like asthma or bronchitis can also cause it.

Precautions

1. If there is choking on account of food etc in the case of infants, give the child many hard slaps on the back between the shoulders. This should shift the obstruction. At times the child may have to hold upside down.
2. In difficult cases an abdominal thrust may have to be given by putting the child one's lap, face away from one's face, and pressing the tips of two fingers of each hand side by side, slightly above the navel, gently but firmly. In all cases see that the air passages of the causality are clear. Put him on his back; turn his head to one side. Remove blood or any other substance from the mouth.

Medicines

1. CICUTA 200 would relax the oesophagus. The spasm will cease and the bone or other matter obstructing the flow of air can be taken out.
2. CARBO-VEG 200 helps in asphyxia by increasing the capacity of the patient to take oxygen and utilize it. It helps even in collapse with cold breath, cold tongue and cold face. In such cases the face goes blue on account of lack of oxygen.

Asthmatic attack

Severe asthmatic attacks cause disproportionate suffering. There is difficulty in breathing. The lungs are full of mucus, which cannot be taken out.

Precautions

1. The patient should be made to sit in an upright position, raise his forearms on some support in front. See that the elbows are spread out in such a way that the chest muscles are not under pressure.
2. The room should be kept warm and moist by the supply of steam from a boiling water cauldron.

Medicines

1. ACONITE 30 and IPECAC 30 should be given alternately every 15 minutes to control the attack. 10 pills of each medicine can be dissolved in half a cup of water and a few sips taken to make a dose, but each time before taking a sip the solution should be stirred well. As soon as the attack is under control, the interval between the doses can be increased to one hour or more.

2. ANTIMONIUM TART 1000 should be given to help the patient take out the mucus from the lungs in case he cannot do so on his own.

❑❑❑

CHAPTER 8

Acne or Pimples

Pimples are very common in young people during their teen years. This condition, which is also known as acne, is apparently due to certain hormone changes in the body. It is particularly prevalent during early adolescence, from 12 to 16 years of age, and is more likely to occur in those who have an oily skin. In the early stages a blackhead or comedone blocks the outlet of an oil gland within the skin. This is not a serious problem, for it leaves no permanent effect.

If the sebaceous duct ruptures and the oily material ooze out between the layers of the skin instead of coming to the surface, there may be a cyst or swelling known as a sebaceous cyst. These are somewhat disfiguring, but not harmless unless they become infected and form small abscesses. When these heal they may leave ugly scars. Severe acne may occur on the shoulders, the back and chest, as well as the face and neck.

Effects of diet: Acne is not caused by diet, but certain foods definitely aggravate this condition, especially in some patients. Rich foods, such as chocolate, nuts, cola drinks, ice-cream, fatty meats, and excessive amount of sugar, all seem to aggravate this condition. Certain drugs, such as those containing bromides and iodides, may also play a part in some people.

Some girls develop one to two pimples just before menstruation. These only last a day or two and are of no consequence. But when acne continues over months or years, it is very distressing, especially to a young woman, and something should definitely be done to clear up the condition. Nervous tension due to family trouble may also play a part in continuing this difficult problem. Even in its mildest form, acne usually persists for a year or more until the hormone system of the body has become fully adjusted.

ACNE ROSACEA: Acne rosacea is an abnormal flushing and irritation of the face and nose. It may also affect the cheeks, chin, and forehead at times. Acne rosacea occurs more frequently in middle-aged people. But there are times when it is also seen in children and young adults, particularly if there has been similar trouble in past generations of their family. Certain substances such as coffee, tea, chocolate, nuts and hot spicy food may be associated with this condition. Alcohol may also bring this on. Some medicines, especially those containing iodides and bromides, are likely to cause these unwanted eruptions on the face. Extremes of heat, cold and wind may also aggravate the affected skin. Nervous tension is often a factor. The condition is really a cosmetic problem, but it is most annoying, though not really serious.

Keep the skin clean by thorough washing two or three times a day with good toilet soap. Warm moist towels applied to the face for ten or fifteen minutes before the treatment will make the removal of blackheads easier. If pus has formed under the skin, be careful not to open the pimple until it is ready to drain. Squeezing and pinching of the skin may extend the inflammation and delay healing, and may also cause scarring of the face.

Avoid all rich foods, excessive amounts of sugar, and particularly chocolate and nuts. Choose a plain, well balanced diet containing plenty of fresh fruits and vegetables. Drink water and fruit juices, but avoids highly sweetened drinks. Extra vitamin A tablets should be added to the diet.

Try to sleep at least eight hours every night. Avoid all strains, and follow the principles of good health, as these are essential for health.

Homoeopathic Medicines

KALI BROMATUM: It produces acne on the face, neck and shoulders. We frequently find acne in Epileptics who have been maltreated by bromides. This remedy is especially adapted to the acne simplex and acne indurate, especially in hyperaesthetics, nervous females. Since Kali bromatum has been found a useful remedy in sexual excesses it will be especially a remedy in acne due to that cause.

SULPHUR: Is perhaps the remedy most often indicated in this affection especially if chronic. The skin is rough and hard and the acne is associated with comedones and constipation; great aggravation from water is the characteristic leading to sulphur in skin affections. Standing is the worst position for Sulphur patients, it is always uncomfortable. It is suited to dirty, filthy people prone to skin affections. When carefully selected remedies fail to act, especially in acute diseases, it frequently arouses the reactionary powers of the organism. Very red lips and face, flushing easily. Often great use in beginning the treatment of chronic cases and finishing the acute ones. Itching, burning of the skin, worse scratching and washing. Skin affections after local medication. Purities, especially from warmth, in evening, often reoccurs in spring time, in damp weather.

NATRUM MUR: It acts especially on the sebaceous glands and is very helpful remedy in acne. Skin is greasy, oily especially on the hairy parts. Dry eruptions especially on the margin of hairy scalp and bends of joints. Face is oily as if greased. Earthy complexion of the face. Patient is irritable and gets into a passion about trifles. Wants to be alone to cry. Tears with laughter. Great weariness and weakness.

PULSATILLA: Pimples after rich food, with diarrhoea, from delayed menses. Acne at puberty. The disposition and mental state are the chief guiding symptoms to the selection of this remedy. The patient seeks the open air; always feel better there, even though he is chilly. Often indicated after abuse of iron tonics.

ANTIMONIUM CRUDUM: Small red pimples on face, acne in drunkards with gastric derangements, thirst and white-coated tongue. Sensitive to cold bathing. Thick, hard, honey coloured scabs. Dry skin. Scaly, pustular eruption with burning and itching, worse at night. Yellow crusted eruption on cheeks and chin. Pimples, pustules and boils on face. Excessive irritability and fretfulness, together with thickly coated white tongue, are true guiding symptoms to many forms of disease calling for this remedy. Cannot bear heat of sun. Heat and cold bathing aggravate all the conditions.

BERBERIS AQUIFOLIUM: It is useful where the skin is rough and the acne persistent. Acne, blotches and pimples. Clears the complexion. Skin is pimply, dry, rough and scaly. Eruption on scalp extending to face and neck.

PHOSPHORUS: Pale sickly complexion, blue rings under eyes. Tearing pains in facial bones; circumscribed redness in one or both cheeks. Little ulcer outside of large ones. It is suited to tall, slender persons, narrow chested, with thin transparent skin, weakened by loss of animal fluids, with great nervous debility and emaciation. Ill effects of iodine and excessive use of salt. Phosphorus irritates, inflames and degenerates mucous membranes, irritates and inflames serous membranes.

□□□

CHAPTER 9

Alcohol - Treatment in Homoeopathy

For ages, man has consumed alcohol to forget his sorrows, to lead him into the realm of happiness. John Keats (1795 -1821), the great romantic English poet, listened to the full-throated music of a nightingale and wanted to become one with that moment of happiness. He thought of taking 'a beaker full of the warm south, of vintage, that has been cooled a long age in the deep delved earth', drinking which he could ' leave the world unseen', and fade away into the dim forest with the singing bird. But Keats was romanticizing the effect of wine on the human mind. A moment later, he decided to give up the idea of taking the assistance of Bacchus and his leopards and switched over to reaching the bird and its music on 'the viewless wings of poesy'. This was definitely a wise decision because the alleged euphoric effect on alcohol is a myth. In fact alcohol dulls the brain and retards its activity.

Alcohol is basically a drug. Man consumes it more than any other drug. No form of alcohol, however mild, whether wine or beer or cider, can do good to the human system and health.

It is fallacy to believe that alcohol stimulates the brain. In reality, alcohol depressed the brain. It slows down various centers of control. When alcohol is swallowed, it goes into the stomach where a fraction of the dose enters the blood stream through the blood vessels of the stomach walls. From the stomach, alcohol has to pass into the small intestine. The carbon dioxide in soda water accelerates this flow of alcohol from the stomach into the intestines. This is what makes whisky and soda more dangerous than whisky and water.

Most of the alcohol that goes into the body is oxidized by the liver and converted into acetic acid, which can be used by the body. But the liver cannot do the job beyond its capacity. As a result, the liver cannot handle any excessive intake of alcohol in a short period of time. Perforce it continues to circulate with the blood stream, affects the brain more and more, and causes intoxication and the resultant aberration in behavior and other problems.

Any person who is fond of alcohol should remember that the liver couldn't process more than a quarter of an ounce of alcohol in an hour. Any dose larger than this puts a burden on the capacity of the liver. In the long run, this damages the liver cells and may lead to cirrhosis of liver, which in turn can be fatal.

The biggest asset of the human body is the brain. Alcohol is one drug, which causes the maximum damage to the brain. Its effects on other organs of the body are via the disorientation of the various parts of the brain. To begin with, alcohol affects parts of the brain, which control thinking and learning. The person who is drinking cannot concentrate, is no longer alert and cannot perform arithmetical exercises as efficiently as a normal person who has not taken alcohol would do. As Thomas Bacon (1512 -1567), the English philosopher and essayist put it, " For when the wine is in, the wit is out".

As the liquor starts having its effect, the human brain is flooded by ideas and images. It is different matter, though important, the coherence is lacking in the ideas and the images are disjointed.

Since ancient times, it has been thought that 'wine maketh glad the heart of man' (The Bible: Psalms104, 15). But in reality, this is a mistaken notion. In the bible itself we find a contradiction: "wine is a mocker, strong drink is raging: and whosoever is deceived thereby is not wise." The second statement is more scientific. The euphoria generated by alcohol is illusory. The blood is warm and so is the skin. It is this warmth, which makes people feel that they have reached the seventh heaven. In reality, the temperature of the body comes down because the heat carried to the skin is soon dissipated by its contact with the air.

It is a fallacy that alcohol improves sexual desire and enjoyment. Make no mistake. Alcohol is no good in adding to sexual enjoyment because sex, to a great extent, is a function of the mind and alcohol dulls the brain. The porter, in William Shakespeare's play 'Mac Beth', puts it succinctly: "it provokes the desire, but it takes away the performance. Therefore much drink may be said to be an equivocator with lechery."

An intake of alcohol leads to frequent urination because it affects a part of the brain, which regulates the functions of the kidney discharging water.

Who does not know that an evening of cozy drinking is followed by a hangover? The random house dictionary defines hangover as the disagreeable physical after effects of drunkenness, usually felt several hours after cessation of drinking." The sufferer feels fatigued on waking up. He has not had enough rest. He would normally have continued drinking late into the night, his awareness of the need to rest and go to sleep having been lost somewhere on the way as a result of the effect of alcohol on the brain. There is severe headache, nausea and indigestion. The tongue is dry, parched like paper on account of an excessive output of urine. The gentleman is thirsty. All this is not a welcome price to pay for the illusory pleasure of an evening of drinking.

Barbiturates and a number of tranquilizers taken in heavy doses after an excessive intake of alcohol can cause death.

Shun alcohol as far as possible. If you just cannot help it, take a moderate quantity at long intervals. Go to bed early as a matter of habit.

When a social drinker cannot cry halt, he is said to be suffering from alcoholism as a disease. The person does not know does not want to know when to stop drinking. He starts drinking when alone and wants to hide his habit from others.

Homoeopathic Medicines

NUX VOMICA: Nux is the great anti - alcoholic remedy. It corresponds to the tremor, to the nervous affections, to the headache, to the bad taste. It also corresponds to delirium tremens, where every little noise frightens and the victim finds no rest in any place, springs up at night and has frightful visions. The tremor is marked with ugliness and irritability and gastric disturbance. It is the right remedy for the acute results of a spree; the morning big head is often large enough for the Nux cap, and the "rich brown" taste corresponds beautifully. It is a remedy to be given while the patient is still under the influence of liquor or any of the stages of alcoholism.

Agaricus will sometimes control the characteristic tremor when Nux fails.

HYOSCYAMUS: When delirium tremens occurs this is usually one of the first remedies indicated. The delirium is constant and loquacious, rarely inflammatory enough for Belladonna or maniacal enough for Stramonium; the pulse is small and quick and compressible, the skin is cold and clammy, the patient is tremulous and picks constantly at objects in the air. Marked sexual excitement desire to expose person and fear of the poison. The visions are those persecution, are terrifying, and the patient makes efforts to escape. Constant insomnia is an excellent indication; outburst of laughter, alternating with weeping may also occur. Dr. Butlet says that for the production of sleep no remedy compares with Hyocyamus in the tincture, five or ten drops in a half glass of water, and teaspoonful doses given half an hourly.

OPIUM: This is a remedy in "old sinners" who have had the delirium tremens over and over again. There is a constant expression of fright or terror, they have visions of animals springing up everywhere, they see ghosts, the sleep in uneasy, the breathing is stertorous. It is especially indicated in those cases stimulating apoplexy. Lachesis has visions of snakes and hideous objects. It has a choking sensation in throat, which awakens suddenly from sleep.

ARSENIC: Has visions of ghosts, with great weakness; diseases from overuse of alcohol; patients must have their accustomed drinks; great tremulousness and nervous weakness. Suicidal tendency, constantly annoyed by bugs and vermin that he sees upon his person and unnecessary tries to brush them off.

BELLADONNA: Has delirium with visions of rats, mice, etc. and so has Calcarea carbonica. Belladonna is easily distinguished from Opium and Calcarea comes in as a last resort after Belladonna and Stramonium have ceased to do well. Aconite also worked well in the acute mania of delirium tremens where the prevailing attitude is fear. Fears darkness, ghosts, with same desire to escape found under Belladonna.

SULPHURIC ACID: This is the remedy for chronic alcoholism. It corresponds to inebriates on their last legs, who are pale and shriveled and cold, whose stomach will not tolerate the slightest amount of food. They cannot drink water unless it will be well whisked. They are quick and hasty in every thing, and have a great and constant craving for brandy. It comes in long after Nux vomica, perhaps after Keely and other cures have failed over and over again. It suits the sour breath and vomiting of alcoholic dyspepsia. It may be given low. "Should it produce a diarrhoea Pulsatilla is the proper anti dote." (Dr. Luther Peck). The constant craving for brandy reminds one of Sulphur, Nux vomica and Arsenicum, all of which craving for spirituous liquors.

CHAPTER 10

Asthma

Asthma is a condition of sudden paroxysmal, expiratory, wheezing dyspnoea caused by an abnormal response of the respiratory center to stimulus causing hyperactivity of the vagal endings in the broncho-constricting muscles resulting in bronchial spasm; with it, hyperaemia of the mucous membrane followed by excessive bronchial secretion is associated.

This is true spasmodic asthma and in this other conditions of periodic expiratory dyspnoea with a different primary factor should not be included.

The disease has in most a family history and is more common in males; sometimes found in young children but more frequently begins in early adult life. Some of these have definite bronchitis also but in the most, the main is paroxysmal bronchospasm no physical sign obtained in the lungs.

The factors concerned in asthma are (i) bronchospasm from causes central and peripheral, (ii) oedema of the bronchial mucous membrane from allergy. Neuropathic predisposition.

The more immediate causes are (i) allergy, (ii) peripheral stimuli from their site of production, grouped as (a) naso-pharyngeal, (b) alimentary, (c) endocrine (d) broncho-pulmonary (iii) constitutional disturbances.

(i) *Allergy:* This is hypersensitiveness to a foreign particle, such as bacterial, animal emanations or vegetable products, chemicals, certain drugs and certain eatables. It is believed to be responsible for bronchospasm.

(ii) Peripheral irritations may be in the nose, inflammation of the mucous membrane, polyps, enlarged tonsils, gastro-intestinal disturbances, uterine or ovarian disorders in the female, bronchopulmonary conditions as emphysema, chronic bronchitis.

(iii) Constitutional disorders such as gout and TB factor.

During an attack the bronchial mucous membrane is swollen and turgid, the bronchial muscles are in spasm and masses of sticky mucus collect in the bronchi. The smaller bronchi and bronchioles are narrowed so that the inspiration is slightly difficult but the expiration is much difficult, the air is retained in the alveoli, which get hyper distended. Afterwards, bronchial secretion begins, the muscle reflex ending in paroxysm. In chronic cases, thickening of the bronchial mucous membrane with eosinophillic infiltration of the basement membrane and peribronchial tissues, eosinophils in the blood, sputum and nasal secretions occur. If the paroxysms are frequently repeated, the lungs become emphysematous and the pulmonary capillary bed is lessened finally right ventricular and general venous stasis follow.

The attack usually begins at the early hours of the morning or soon after exposure to the allergen. There may be some warnings as restlessness, mental exaltation or depression, sneezing or coryza, flatulence, the patient if asleep suddenly wakes up with a sense of suffocation. Dyspnoea increases and he sits up in the bed panting for breath, head low and the elbows on the knees frequently using the accessory muscles of respiration also. But the respiratory rate is not increased. There is often irritable cough with wheezing in the chest. As the expectoration becomes free, the attack comes to an end. Large quantity of urine may be passed and the patient goes to sleep.

The chest is full with very little inspiratory expansion and in a severe case, with sucking in of the supraclavicular and subcostal regions and is hyper resonant on percussion; the inspiration is short and laboured and the expiration is noisy and prolonged. On auscultation, the breath sound is feeble, and later, copious bubbling rales are heard. Pulse is often quick and feeble and systolic BP may be lowered. Jugular veins may be prominent.

Sputum often shows many eosinophils in the mucus. The attack may recur nearly at the same time every night and continue for weeks or months. There may be periods of intermission tends to be progressively short. In a long-standing case, lungs get emphysematous, chronic bronchitis is superadded and ultimately right heart failure comes in.

CHRONIC ASTHMA: If the attacks are repeated for years, certain peculiarities appear. The patient is thin, long neck, and barrel shaped chest with a forward stoop and he is easily out of breath: a chronic cough is often present. He develops anxiety neurosis being always apprehensive of a paroxysm.

Diagnosis is made from family history, personal history, and onset at an early age. Type of cough, expectoration, the blood and sputum shows eosinophils.

Homoeopathic Medicines

IPECACHUANA: There is great anxiety and weight about the chest; sudden wheezing, dsypnoea, threatening suffocation, aggravated by motion, the cough causes gagging and vomiting. The cough is constant, the chest seems full of phlegm yet nothing is expectorated and the extremities are covered with cold perspiration. The expiration is difficult; vomiting when it occurs is apt to relieve the attack. Yearly attacks of difficult shortness of breathing. Continued sneezing, coryza, wheezing cough. Cough incessant and violent, with every breath. Suffocative cough; child becomes stiff and blue in the face. Bleeding from lungs, with nausea, feeling of constriction. Hoarseness especially at the end of cold.

ARSENIC ALB: The attack occurs after midnight. The patient has great deal of anguish and restlessness; he cannot lie down for fear of suffocation. There is anxiety and general sweat, and if the patient drowses off he is awakened with burning pain and soreness in the chest. It is especially a remedy for chronic cases. The asthma of Arsenic is accompanied by great debility and burning in the chest and is useful in anaemic persons. Its range of action upon these tissues and organs is from simple irritation to total destruction. Weakness, emaciation, irritable stomach, intense thirst, sharp, shooting pains ameliorated by heat are some of the symptoms of the arsenic alb. Cough is worse after midnight; worse lying down on back. Haemoptysis with pain between shoulders; burning heat all over. Cough dry as from sulphur fumes, after drinking. Thirst for small quantities of water at small intervals.

NATRUM SULPH: Its general symptoms are worse on change to damp weather. There is moist asthma, with a great deal of rattling in the chest. The symptoms of looseness of bowels after each attack have been found in most cases. The attacks generally comes on about 4 or 5 o' clock in the morning with cough and rising of glary slime; expectoration greenish and copious. An important symptom present is that the patient must sit up and hold the chest with the hands during the attack. Cough with thick ropy, greenish expectoration; chest feels all gone. Constant desire to take deep breath, asthma in children. Pain through lower left chest. Every fresh cold brings on attack of asthma.

ANTIMONIUM TART: There is presence of fine mucus rales throughout the chest. The chest seems full of phlegm, with inability to expectorate it. There is great dsypnoea, the patient must sit up, and there are suffocative attacks coming on at about 3 o'clock in the morning. There is difficulty in the expectoration. It is especially adapted to the extremes of life. The sensation that the patient cannot air enough is the characteristic symptom. Burning sensation in chest, which ascends to throat, rapid, short, difficult breathing seems as if he would suffocate. Bronchial tubes overloaded with mucus. Cough excited by eating with pain in the chest and larynx. Oedema and impending paralysis of the lungs. Pulse rapid, weak and trembling, dizziness with cough. Dsypnoea relieved by eructation. Cough and dsypnoea better by lying on right side.

CHAPTER 11

Baldness

Partial or complete loss of hair on the scalp is rather common among them. This is more or less to be expected in the female. Premature baldness is a tendency in certain families. Thinning of the hair is often seen in older women, but complete baldness in the female is fortunately rare. Temporary baldness may occur following a fever or some prolonged illness. The hair usually returns after the patient has recovered from the illness.

Sudden loss of the hair in certain areas, a condition called alopecia areata, may sometimes follows extreme nervous shock. This may clear up in a few weeks, although sometimes it will recur. In females excessive hair loss is seen after delivery and during lactation. This is only due to hormonal changes in the body and due to suckling of the milk by the child. This disappears after the child stops weaning. It is not a permanent problem. In children falling of hair occurs due to many reasons such as severe headache, dim eyesight, after a prolonged illness, use of different shampoos and soaps, after a severe head injury and a familial tendency. Generally it is observed that if the parents have thin hair and early loss of hair in their life so is their children.

Many people use various shampoos and creams to prevent hair loss but with no gain. Homoeopathy has a very good treatment for hair loss. Some of the important medicines indicated in the hair loss are given below:

Homoeopathic Medicines

NATRUM MUR: It has the symptoms of easy falling out of the hair; it falls out when touched or combed. This is frequently seen in nursing women. Hair becomes thin. During confinement hair fall off from the genitals. Marked debility and weariness. Chronic disease resulting in depression. Irritable. Effects of fright, grief, anger. Dry eruptions; crusty eruptions on the margin of the scalp. Eczema of the scalp. Anaemic headache of schoolgirls. Chronic headache, semi lateral, congestive, from sunrise to sunset, with pale face, nausea and vomiting. The patient requiring this remedy is melancholic, hypochondriac, sad and hopeless about the future, easily angered, consolation aggravates. There is emaciation and prematurely aged look.

PHOSPHORUS: Bald spots on the head, which are dry and scaly. Dandruff, roots of hair get gray and the hair comes out in bunches. The head sweats easily. The most important remedy in alopecia areata. Pale sickly complexion, blue rings under eyes. Phosphorus irritates, inflames and degenerates mucous membranes, irritates and inflames serous membranes. It is suited to tall, slender persons, narrow chested, with thin transparent skin, weakened by loss of animal fluids, with great nervous debility and emaciation. Chronic congestion of head, brain fag with coldness of occiput. Vertigo with faintness. Itching of scalp, dandruff, falling out of hair in large bunches.

PHOSPHORIC ACID: Falling of hair from general debility. Pain in the temples as if crushed together. Hair gray early in life; falls out. Dull headache after coition; form eyestrain. Vertigo towards evening, when standing or walking. Hair thins out, gray early. It is mostly suitable to young people who grow rapidly and who are overexerted mentally or physically. Blue rings around the eyes.

FLOURIC ACID: Alopecia, caries of skin. Pressure on sides of head from within outward. Falling of hair from syphilis. Profuse, sour, offensive perspiration. Patient is worse from warmth, in the morning, warm drinks. Better by cold, while walking.

SEPIA: It has loss of hair after chronic headache. Weakness, yellow complexion, bearing down sensation is the most important guiding symptoms of this remedy. Feels cold even in a warm room. Vertigo with sensation of something rolling round in head. Stinging pain from within outward and upward mostly left, or in forehead, with nausea vomiting; worse indoors and when lying on painful side. Roots of hair sensitive. Pimples on forehead near hair.

LYCOPODIUM: Premature baldness and gray hair. Great falling out of hair. Eczema; moist oozing behind ears. Tearing pains in occiput; better fresh air. Pain in temples as if they were screwed against each other. Vertigo in morning on rising. Pressing headache on vertex; worse from 4 to 8 p.m. and from lying down or stooping, if no eating regularly. Shakes head without apparent cause. Best adapted to persons intellectually keen but of weak muscular power. Lycopodium patient is thin, withered, full of gas and dry.

Lacks vital heat; has poor circulation, cold extremities. Sensitive to noise and odors.

ARSENIC ALB: Bald spots near the forehead; the scalp is covered with dry scales. The patient has great deal of anguish and restlessness; he cannot lie down for fear of suffocation. Headache relieved by cold other symptoms worse. Head is in constant motion. Face is swollen, pale, yellow, cachetic, sunken cold and covered with sweat. Scalp itches intolerable; circular patches of bare spots; rough dirty, sensitive and covered with dry scales; nightly burning and itching; dandruff. Scalp very sensitive cannot brush hair.

GRAPHITES: Humid, itching eruption on hairy scalp, emitting a fetid odor. Headache in morning on waking, mostly on one side, with inclination to vomit. Sensation of cobweb on forehead. It is especially suited to patients who are rather stout, of fair complexion; with tendency to skin affections and constipation, fat, chilly and costive, with delayed menstrual history, take cold easily.

NITRIC ACID: Sensation of a band around head. Headache from pressure of hat; full feeling; worse from street noises. Hair falls out. Scalp sensitive. Black pores on face, papules worse on forehead.

□□□

CHAPTER 12

Bed Wetting

By the time a child reaches the age of two he can usually keep himself dry during the day. However, it may be another year or more before he can keep dry all through the night. Even then, the best-trained child may fail to live up to expectations on certain occasions when he is highly excited.

Older boys and girls may also have occasional problems at night, especially when sleeping in a strange bed after a highly exciting evening.

The bladder is emptied unconsciously especially during sleep at night; may be associated with enlarged tonsils, thyroid deficiency, phimosis, intestinal worms, blanitis or vulvitis also sometimes pyelitis, cystitis, oxaluria even minor epilepsy.

There are many causes for this condition, ranging all the way from simple neglect of the calls of nature to degenerative changes in the spinal cord. The condition is found in all classes and at all ages. Nocturnal bedwetting is very common in weak, neurotic children. The next most numerous class is that of women who have born children and who have passed the fiftieth milestone. A laugh, a sneeze, a fright and the urine spurt from the bladder. Probably this is want of proper adjustment of the function of the nervous mechanism of the sphincter and the detrusor and the former fails to inhibit the later.

Here are some tips to help overcome bedwetting:

1. Don't be overanxious about this problem. Making an issue of it may only enhance the problem. Try to keep the child relaxed even if he is a little slow in outgrowing this habit.

2. Reduce the amount of fluid just before the child goes to bed. Don't be unreasonable, especially on a hot night, for the more concentrated urine may be irritating the child and causing him to lose control of his bladder during sleep.
3. Be sure to reward him in some suitable manner when he succeeds in keeping dry at night. Do not punish him when he fails, but when he succeeds give him some privilege, which he values highly.
4. Take him to the toilet before you go to bed yourself, especially if this is a frequent problem.
5. Give your child a happy home of which he can be truly proud. Try to remove all friction within the family. This may help to solve not only the bed-wetting but all other nervous problems as well.

Besides these tips treatment for bedwetting in homoeopathy is given as under:

Homoeopathic Medicines

NUX VOMICA: It affects the urinary organs powerfully. It affects the lower part of the spine; there is irritability at the neck of the bladder. Incontinence of urine. There are frequent efforts to urinate and burning and tearing pains accompany these; the urine passes in drops. Paralysis of the bladder and there is dribbling of the urine. Cystitis, with painful urging calls for this remedy. The straining is violent at times and the urine is dark with red brick sediment, or bloody or mixed with tenacious mucus. Irritable bladder; from spasmodic sphincter. While urinating itching in urethra and pain in neck of bladder.

CAUSTICUM: In paralytic states of the bladder it is the first remedy to be thought of. It is one of the great remedies in enuresis and its characteristic symptoms are involuntary micturition at night in sleep, when coughing, sneezing or blowing the nose, showing a weakness of the sphincter. There is difficulty in passing the last few drops of urine; the patient has to wait a long time before it starts and during the act it passes very slowly showing a weakness of the whole muscular system of the bladder. Nocturnal wetting of the bed in children, occurring during the first sleep at night. Paralysis of the bladder after labor also calls for this remedy. There are excessive deposits of urates in urine. It is also a useful remedy for retention of urine after surgical operations. Loss of sensibility on passing urine.

SEPIA: It is the remedy for wetting the bed at night during the first sleep. It has reddish clay colored sediment adhering to the vessel, sediment of red sand. Offensive urine. This is a very useful remedy in renal colic and gravel.

The patient has to micturate every few minutes, during which he wrings his hands and groans with pain. Nausea is often present. The quantity of sand deposited is very large. It is often indicated in cystitis with a constant desire to urinate and dragging in the bladder.

CANTHARIS: It is the first remedy required for a urinary difficulty. There is persistent and violent urging to urinate, with great tenesmus; the urine is passed through the urethra, burning is very intense. There is aching in the small of back. It is often indicated in acute cystitis; gravel and uretheritis, important symptoms being the burning and the tenesmus of the bladder; haematuria also calls for this remedy. There is constant urging to urinate, even small amount of urine in the bladder bringing the urging, which is accompanied by the terrible distress at the neck of the bladder. In the region of the kidneys there is cutting pain, which extends to the abdomen, the bladder and urethra. The pain is aggravated immediately following urination. The urine itself under Cantharis is of a deep red color, deposits sediment of mucus and often contains fibrinous cast.

EQISETUM: There is pain in the bladder as if too full, not relieved by micturition; the constant desire to urinate is not even relieved by copious urination. The urine is scanty; high colored and contains much mucus. Difficulty in beginning to urinate, strains a great deal, scanty urine. It has proved useful in enuresis with marked vesicle irritation. It is indicated in dsyuria of children, the pain being worse after urinating. Urine flows only drop-by-drop. Sharp, burning, cutting pain in urethra while urinating. Incontinence in children with dreams of nightmares when passing urine. Incontinence in old women also with involuntary stools. Retention and dsyuria during pregnancy and after delivery.

APIS MELLIFICA: The most important symptoms for Apis in urinary infections are scanty or suppressed urine, drowsiness, and oedema in various parts, thirstlessness and suffocation on lying down. The urine is dark, highly albuminous, and contains casts. In difficult micturition of Apis is a useful remedy. It has a frequent desire, with the passage of few drops at a time. There is great irritation at the neck of the bladder and incontinence of urine. Burning and soreness when urinating. Urine is suppressed loaded with casts; frequent and involuntary, stinging pain and strangury. Last drops burn and smart. Swelling or puffing up of various parts, oedema, red rosy hue, stinging pains, soreness, intolerance of heat, and slightest touch, and afternoon aggravation are some of the important guiding symptoms.

CHAPTER 13

Bronchitis

Bronchitis may be defined as a distressing and often serious type of inflammation affecting the windpipe, or bronchial tubes, in the chest. There are two types of bronchitis:

1. Acute Bronchitis
2. Chronic Bronchitis

Acute bronchitis: In acute bronchitis the larynx, trachea and bronchial tubes are acutely inflamed. The tissues are swollen because of irritation; large amount of mucus is secreted and poured into the bronchial tubes to protect the inflamed mucous membrane. Unless this thick, sticky material is removed, it may obstruct the windpipe, causing more severe diseases like atelactasis and pneumonia. The common cold is probably the most frequent cause of acute bronchitis.

During the acute stage of bronchitis there is usually a high fever and some difficulty in breathing. There is a constant cough. Hoarseness may also be present and some pain in the chest. Difficulty in breathing continues until the inflammation has decreased. And thick secretions have removed. Chilliness is present with internal coldness, also cold hands and feet, rawness beneath the sternum, some tightness and oppression of the chest, cough may be dry, hard, ringing, expulsive, paroxysmal, tearing which leaves great soreness under the sternum. After few days the cough, which was at first dry, becomes moist and is accompanied by slight expectoration of mucus and occasionally some blood. As the amount of expectoration increases all the other symptoms decreases, and then in turn abnormal secretion and expectoration also decreases at the end of 7 to 10 days.

Chronic bronchitis: It is of long duration. This condition arises from sinusitis, nasal drip, or infected tonsils and adenoids. In chronic bronchitis permanent change may have occurred in the lungs such as pulmonary fibrosis, emphysema and other serious complications.

Normally the lungs are very elastic and flexible. It is their function to expand and contract within the chest as we breathe in and out. Any chronic inflammation of the lungs, such as fibrosis or scarring, interferes with the normal movement of the lungs so that the air cannot be inhaled and exhaled freely. In asthmatic patients and those suffering from tuberculosis or congestive heart failure the situation becomes worse. Severe coughing may produce blood as well as copious mucus filled with pus and bacteria. This will lead to Bronchopneumonia a more serious condition.

Those who suffer from chronic bronchitis should stop smoking and remain in a smoke free atmosphere as much as possible. Such patients should avoid heavy exercise. They should adopt the occupations that do not require heavy breathing. As far as possible they should avoid cold draughts of air for these always bring on a paroxysm of coughing. The patient should follow a good, well balanced diet and take extra vitamins to aid in the healing of the inflamed tissues.

Homoeopathic Medicines

ACONITE: In Aconite the causes for the Bronchitis may be checked perspiration, exposure to cold, drafts or dry, cold winds. The attack comes on with marked chilliness, often chill followed by a high temperature, dry hot skin, a very rapid pulse, a dry rough cough, constriction and tightness of the chest, anxiety, fear of death, great restlessness and intense thirst. Aconite will often prevent the development of a chronic bronchitis. Constant pressure in left chest. Larynx sensitive. Hot feeling in lungs. Blood comes up with hawking. Tingling in chest after cough. Shortness of breath. Child grasps at throat every time he coughs. Very sensitive to inspired air.

BELLADONNA: It suits cases of bronchitis with a violent fever, short dry, and continually distressing cough worse at night and on lying down, where the breathing is irregular and hurried, no expectoration, or, if present it is blood streaked, fullness in chest without any pain. The skin is hot and inclined to moisture. The patient is drowsy, the patient does not sleep. Cough is spasmodic and the child cries after each paroxysm. Larynx feel sore. Cheyne-strokes breathing. Cough with pain in left hip. Barking cough, whooping cough, with pain in stomach before attack, with expectoration of blood. Larynx very painful. Stitches in chest when coughing. Respiration oppressed, quick, unequal.

BRYONIA: This remedy is indicated in pure Bronchitis, very frequently. It is a good service when the cough is severe it hurts the head and distant parts of the body. The patient presses his hands and on the sides of the chest while coughing relieves the pain. There is a great pressure on the sternum; dyspnoea and a dry cough which starts from the stomach. After a meal it gets worse, a little expectoration. The cough is the result of an irritation in the larger bronchi than in the finer tubes, hacking produces sore spots in the trachea and chest. Stitching pain in the sides, indicate Bryonia. Coming into the warm room from the cold air aggravates the cough. It is the best remedy after Aconite, which is cold on the chest. Pulsatilla can be taken if the expectoration becomes copious, loose, thick and muco-purulent. If it is accompanied by nausea and vomiting of mucus, Ipecachuana is indicated. Chellidonium is an excellent medicine in a capillary bronchitis following measeals and whooping cough.

PHOSPHORUS: It is suitable to sub-acute and in lingering case in delicate, tall, slender or overgrown. It suits non-resistant individuals. Cough with pain, suffocative pressure in the upper part of the chest with constriction of larynx, hoarseness mucous rales mucous sputum and bloody and having a taste of salty or sweetish. Patient gets relief after sleep. The respiration is embraced and its tendency towards pneumonia. In the supra-sternal fossa Rumex has a tingling; change in breathing causes cough. It must breathe in warm air so that cough can be avoided. The cough is worse after meals Phosphorus is indicated. Symptoms are rawness and soreness of the chest; cough is also worse going into the fresh air being a reverse of Bryonia.

ANTIMONIUM TART: This remedy corresponds to two stages of bronchitis, an early one and a late one. In the beginning of capillary bronchitis in young infants, or in old people, this remedy stands most prominent. There are sub-crepittent rales through out the chest. The cough is loose, and there is no phlegm. In children the cough is infrequent, and the child is drowsy, the respiration is superficial, requiring labored efforts of the respiratory muscles and vomiting of food and mucus may be present. With Antimonium tart there is great oppression of breathing, worse towards morning, compelling the patient to sit up to breathe. There are also sharp, stitching pains and high fever, perhaps it corresponds more to the catarrhal form than it does to the croupous form. There is one peculiar symptom, the patient feels sure that the next cough will raise the mucus, but it does not

IPECACUANHA: In case of this medicine the rales are louder and coarser, there is much coughing, and the patient expectorates little mucus. It is one of the best remedies in the capillary bronchitis of infants, prostration is less marked. There is great accumulation of mucus, spasmodic cough, nausea and difficulty in breathing. Dsypnoea; constant constriction in chest. Yearly attacks of difficult shortness of breathing. Cough incessant and violent with every breath. Bleeding from lungs, with nausea; feeling of constriction, rattling cough. Hoarseness especially at the end of cold. Complete aphonia.

KALI BI: Expectoration is tough, tenacious, and glutinous. It can be drawn out in long strings. Hughes considers it useful when bronchitis lingers long in sub-acute condition. The expectoration may also be bluish lumps, and the cough is especially troublesome towards morning, the tightness seems to be at the epigastria. Voice hoarse worse in the evening. Profuse yellow expectoration, very glutinous and sticky, coming out in long, stringy and very tenacious mass. True membranous croup, extending to larynx and nares. Cough with pain in sternum extending to shoulders; worse when undressing. Pain at bifurcation of trachea on coughing from midsternum to back.

❑❑❑

CHAPTER 14

Cirrhosis of the Liver

It may be defined as a chronic condition of the liver in which there is an increase of the connective tissue, a decrease in its size, and a degeneration of the parenchyma.

Alcohol is the most common cause of the cirrhosis of liver. Alcohol reaches the liver through blood stream. Other causes may include improperly prepared foods, poisonous substances, drugs like arsenic, phosphorus, the infectious diseases like syphilis and obstruction of the bile ducts.

Cirrhosis of the liver produced by alcohol abuse is known as portal cirrhosis where as cirrhosis caused by some obstruction such as a stone in the common duct or some narrowing of the bile duct leading from the liver to the small intestine is called as Biliary cirrhosis.

There are two conditions of a cirrhotic liver:

1. Atrophic cirrhosis
2. Fatty cirrhosis.

Atrophic cirrhosis: In this condition the size is reduced to half, sometimes to a third its normal size. The liver becomes firm and hard. It is rough, granular and nodular. The cut surface shows grayish-white patches surrounded by yellow patches. The hepatic cells and portal vein are compressed and the circulation interfered with or completely cut off.

Fatty cirrhosis: In this cirrhosis the connective tissue is greatly increased, making the liver large, smooth or slightly angular. The fat is greatly increased, resembling a fatty liver. The circulation is interrupted with as in the atrophic form. The capsule is thickened and opaque and is adherent to the peritoneum by bands and patches. Along with the peritoneum spleen, stomach and intestines are also affected by catarrh.

In Hanot's hypertrophic liver the size is much more increased and the liver cells are enlarged and contain several nuclei. The connective tissue is also greatly increased in this variety.

The patient at first may present with anorexia, belching, bad taste, nausea, pressure in epigastrium, and tenderness in the region of the liver, dsypnoea and hepatic colic.

Other symptoms which are present includes a full red tongue, constipation at times, diarrhoea, constipation and diarrhoea may alternate with each other, hemorrhages from any part of the gastrointestinal tract, enlargement of the liver, emaciation, jaundice of the skin, having a dirty, muddy colour, oedema of the feet, legs, beneath the eyes and about the genitals. The urine is often high coloured, loaded with urea, some bile and if the kidneys are involved albumin and casts is present in the urine. Temperature may be normal or subnormal, rarely elevated. So called "spiders" are seen on the face, neck, and arms and trunk. These are hair like, reddish markings in the skin somewhat resembling small spiders. As the disease continues the abdomen becomes bloated and swollen, the mind is clouded, and there may be considerable bleeding from the stomach.

Homoeopathic Medicines

NUX VOMICA: It is the most frequently indicated remedies. It is mainly a remedy to antidote the effects of alcohol. The liver is swollen hard and sensitive to the touch and pressure of clothing. This the first remedy in the cirrhosis of liver. Colic may be present. Jaundice induced by the anger, from abuse of quinine. Liver engorged with stitches and soreness. Colic with upward pressure, causing short breathe and desire for stool. Weakness of abdominal ring region. Alternate constipation and diarrhoea after the abuse of purgatives. Diarrhoea with jaundice. Bruised soreness of abdominal walls.

LYCOPODIUM: Liver sensitive. Brown spots on abdomen. Desire for sweet things. Aversion to bread, etc. after eating pressure in stomach, with bitter taste in mouth. The region of the liver is sensitive to touch and there is a feeling of tension in it, a feeling as if a cord were tied about the waist. Cirrhosis. Fullness in the stomach after eating a small quantity. There is apt to be weight and aching in the liver, he can lie on that side, but no turning to the left side, the liver seems to pull and draw. Lycopodium is more useful than any other remedy in old hepatic congestions. Pain in right side and back from congestion will often lead to this remedy.

CARBO VEG: Boericke says: "Disintegration and imperfect oxidization is the keynote of this remedy." Lack of vitality, the coldness and weakness, the extreme exhaustion is prominent symptoms. There is great flatulence in the upper part of the abdomen. Pain in the liver, stomach and abdomen due to distension is always present. Carbo veg is most useful when the disease is of some infectious origin. Pain as if from lifting a weight; colic from riding in a carriage. Cannot bear tight clothing around waist and abdomen. Crampy pains forcing the patient to bend double. Nausea in the morning. Burning in stomach, extending to back and along spine.

ARSENIC ALB: It also acts upon all tissues of the alimentary tract. There is diarrhoea. It acts rapidly and violently. Burning is the ranking sensation. Eating and drinking, especially anything cold aggravates the pain and cause vomiting; rapid emaciation results from in ability of retaining the food. The Arsenic patient is always fearful of the outcome of his condition. Great thirst drinks much but little at a time. Nausea, retching, vomiting after eating or drinking anxiety in pit of stomach. Vomiting of blood, bile, green mucous, or brown black mixed with blood. Gastralgia from slightest food or drink. Dyspepsia from vinegar, acids, ice cream and tobacco. Ill effects of vegetable diet, melons and watery fruits generally.

ARGENTUM NITRICUM: It is an excellent remedy to control gastric conditions, which may cause or may be caused by cirrhosis. The nausea, vomiting of glassy mucus shows inflammation and ulceration, the enormous distention, the soreness and tenderness, the offensive green, chopped stools containing blood and mucus are all important symptoms pointing to this remedy. The nervous symptoms are also prominent. There is also a painful swelling of the pit of the stomach; stomach distended by gas with frequent eructation's. In addition to the above nausea, wretching and vomiting is also present. The vomited material staining the cloth black. With the vomiting, which is sometimes mucous, we often find a green mucous stool and occasionally, bloody stools. Complaints are aggravated from pressure, from deep inspiration, from eating or drinking and better by eructating gas, from vomiting. The sensations are gripping with burning; gnawing; stinging ulcerative aggravated by touch and deep inspiration; burning; twisting and soreness. The pains extend from the stomach to the back, chest, shoulders, and down the abdomen.

CHAPTER 15

Common Cold

Although the common cold affects all parts of the body, it usually begins in the nose and throat. Colds are so common we hardly give them a second thought, yet they can be rather serious. Most colds are due to virus infections of one type or another. Unfortunately, none of these viruses are susceptible to our present antibiotic medicines. Adenoviruses produce the more serious type of colds, and they are often followed by tonsillitis and sore throat even virus pneumonia, particularly in children. Sometimes the membranes of the eyes are also involved.

The common cold is the most prevalent of all diseases known to man. The average person seems to have two or three colds a year. The condition is highly contagious. When one member of the family has a cold, the others are very likely to have one within a few days.

What makes a person susceptible to a cold? Probably his lowered resistance is a chief factor. Allergic disorders of the nose and throat also make a person more susceptible to colds and other virus infections. Chilling of the body does seem to play a part, particularly in those whose resistance is already weak. Lack of sleep may be another factor.

Any person may carry the cold virus. However, children under six years of age seem readily to pass the infection from one to another, and soon all the family is involved. Colds are always more serious in the younger children.

Congestion of the nasal passages is usually the first sign of cold. The patient may have frequent sneezing and a severe, throbbing headache. There may be a thin, watery discharge from the nose, requiring the use of many handkerchiefs. The eyes may be red or irritated. Usually there is some rise in temperature, preceded by chilly feelings. The patient may complain of a sore throat and have some difficulty in swallowing. Hoarseness, or laryngitis, indicates that the infection has reached the vocal cords, and the patient may now have to talk in whispers. Later there may be a deep cough, due to bronchitis. This is a much more complication.

Homoeopathic Medicines

ACONITE: When the attack comes on suddenly after an exposure to a cold, dry wind, with chilliness, followed by fever, Aconite will be the remedy. It should be administered just as soon as the patient realizes that he is taking cold. There is as yet no discharge, but from the congestion the nose is swollen, hot, dry and stopped up, and this stoppage is apt to change from side to side; there is tingling and burning in the nose and a throbbing frontal headache; there may be sneezing also. These symptoms are all better in the open air. There is great restlessness, tossing about, anxiety and fear of death. There is suddenness of onset of the symptoms and especially in young and plethoric persons who are full of life and vigour. High fever proceeded by a distinct chill; the pulse is full, hard and tense; a history of exposure may also be taken into consideration; dry cold winds.

ARSENIC ALB: It is especially useful in winter colds where there is a thin, watery discharge from the nostrils which excoriates the upper lip, yet in spite of this fluent discharge the nose feels stopped up. There is dull, frontal headache and sneezing, photophobia, the sneezing does not relieve in the slightest and the irritation continues as before and is worse on going into the open air. Burning and bleeding. Acne of nose. The Arsenic patient is always fearful of the outcome of his condition. Great thirst drinks much but little at a time. Debility, exhaustion and restlessness with nightly aggravation are the leading indications for this remedy. Great exhaustion after the slight exertion. The attack occurs after midnight.

ALLIUM CEPA : It is one of the best remedies for cold in the head. The discharge is profuse, thin and acrid, with great smarting in the nose and eyes. There is profuse lacrymation, which is bland. The edges of the eyelids burn and the eyes are red and sensitive to light. The nasal discharge is thin and flows constantly, excoriates the upper lip, and there is prolonged sneezing. The discharge ceases when the patient goes into the open air, but returns when entering a warm room again. It is a drug which should be given early, and if there be a splitting laryngeal cough, causing the patient to wince and crouch it is indicated. Feeling of a lump at the root of nose. Fluent coryza with headache, cough and hoarseness.

GELSEMIUM: It is not indicated in the early stage of the cold in the head. Fullness of the head, hot fever and chilliness as if a cold were coming on. The patient is dull and weak, chills run up and down the back, with a watery, excoriating, or bland discharge from the nose and sneezing. There is also a marked inclination in the patient to hug the fire. Cold brought on by warm relaxing weather indicate Gelsemium, hence it seems to be, most useful in spring and summer weather. There is a predisposition to take cold on any change of weather. It has been extremely useful in influenza with fever. Sneezing fullness at the root of nose. Headache preceded by blindness better by profuse urination. Wants to have head raised on pillow. Swelling of turbinate. Dryness of nasal fossae. Acute coryza, with dull headache and fever. Watery excoriating discharge. Neuralgia of face. Dusky hue of face with vertigo and dim vision.

NUX VOMICA: Nux vomica has colds caused by cold weather, with a dry, stuffed up nose and rough, scrappy throat. The first stage of ordinary cold in the head may be cured by Nux Vomica, when it is brought on by damp, cold weather, or from sitting on damp, cold steps, associated with sneezing and stuffed up feeling in the nose. The nose is dry, there is very little discharge, the eyes are watery and there is scraping in the throat, and dullness and oppression about the front sinuses; it should be given as soon as dryness and tickling in the nose begins; the nasal passages are alternately free and obstructed. These symptoms are worse in a warm room and better in the open air. It is of little use when the cold is fully developed. Nose is stuffed up at night. Odours tend to produce fainting. Coryza fluent in daytime; stuffed up at night and outdoors; or alternates between nostrils. Bleeding in morning. Acrid discharge, but with stuffed up feeling. Tickling after waking in the morning. Sensation of roughness, tightness and tension.

NATRUM MUR: Colds with watery, transparent discharges causing vesicular eruptions about mouth and nose, which burst and leave thin crusts and scabs. Running colds with watery, clear, frothy discharge, worse on going into air and on exertion; great dryness of posterior nares. There is entire loss of taste. Dropping of mucus from nasopharynx in the morning. It also removes the tendency to take cold. Violent, fluent coryza lasting from one to three days, then changing into stoppage of nose; making breathing difficult. Discharge thin and watery, like raw white of egg. Violent sneezing coryza. Infallible for stopping a cold commencing with sneezing. Internal soreness of nose.

DULCAMARA: Dry coryza renewed by slightest exposure, worse after getting wet, in the open air and at night. It suits especially torpid phlegmatic constitutions, those who take cold when the weather changes to a lower temperature, and so it becomes of great use in nasal catarrhs and influenza of autumn. Colds, which come on from change of weather and gradually involve the whole respiratory tract, may indicate Dulcamara. "Cold sores" may accompany the colds. Dry coryza. Complete stoppage of nose. Thick yellow mucus, bloody crusts. Profuse coryza. Wants nose kept warm, least cold air stops the nose. Coryza of the newborn.

MERCURIUS: There is profuse coryza, which extends to the frontal sinuses burning in eyes and nose, acrid discharge, violent sneezing, and tendency to perspiration, which aggravates. When a cold begins with coryza, mercurius is a valuable remedy. Mercurius is especially aggravated in damp weather and the coryza is worse by heat of stove or room, nose is sore; wiping nose is painful. Much sneezing. Sneezing in sunshine. Nostrils raw and ulcerated; nasal bones swollen. Yellow-green, foetid, puslike discharge. Coryza; acrid discharge, but too thick to run down the lip; worse warm room. Pain and swelling of nasal bones, and caries, with greenish foetid ulceration. Nosebleed at night. Copious discharge of corroding mucus. Coryza, with sneezing; sore, raw, smarting sensation; worse, damp weather, profuse fluent.

❑❑❑

CHAPTER 16

Constipation

Constipation means difficult or infrequent passage of the feces. In some cases it is due to mechanical obstruction of the intestines, such as cancer, diverticulitis, or perhaps to some functional cause, such as an irritable colon discussed above. In most cases there is no actual obstruction.

Many elderly people suffer from constipation; probably they do not take sufficient fluid. They may think they are drinking enough, but careful observation may reveal that they are having only two or three glasses of liquid a day. For normal bowel habits, one should drink from six to eight glasses of fluid each day.

Sometimes constipation results from ignoring the normal call of nature. Many people suffering from constipation become dependent upon laxatives in early childhood. This is most unfortunate, for it means that the child may be dependent on drugs for the rest of his life. As far as possible do not use an enema on a child unless absolutely necessary. Laxatives and enemas are only for unusual conditions. Nature will provide for the normal needs of the body.

Constipation can also result from spasm of a small segment of the sigmoid colon. It should be recalled that motility, even normally, is weak in the large intestine, so that even a slight degree of spasm is often capable of causing serious constipation. After the constipation has continued for several days and excessive feces have accumulated above the spastic sigmoid colon, excessive colonic secretions often lead to a day or so of diarrhoea.

The diet should be rich in fruits and vegetables, for these are natural laxatives. The patient should have regular meals and avoid nervous tension. He should sleep at least 8 hours a night and take regular exercise. Many cases of constipation are relieved by the use of prune juice, figs, bananas, or other natural laxatives. Sensible habits of living, plus 6 - 8 glasses of water per day and a reasonable amount of exercise will cure most people of constipation.

Homoeopathic Medicines

NUX VOMICA: Perhaps no remedy in the Materia Medica is oftener prescribed for anything than is Nux Vomica for constipation. Nux Vomica has peculiar and characteristic indications for constipation, and when prescribed upon these indications it will cure every time. Nux Vomica is often prescribed when these indications are not present, does not much good; in this class of cases there will almost invariably be present one of the great clinical indications of the remedy. And that is, its value in antidoting purgative medicines. Nux vomica has been given to antidote the effects of drastic medicines. Nux is the fact that while prescribed low, as in the tincture, it will frequently relieve constipation, but to cure it, the drug must be given in much higher potency. Hydrastis is another remedy that is sometimes useful after the abuse of purgatives, laxatives, cathartics and their like. Hydrastis has a symptom, however, which is quite characteristic that is sinking, gone feeling at epigastrium, which Nuxvomica does not have to any extent. The constipation of Nux Vomica is usually of the kind induced by lazy habits, inattention to nature's calls in the first place, want of exercise, sedentary habits and a sluggish condition of the whole system. It is not only due to inactivity of the intestines, but to irregularity of the peristaltic actions, giving rise to the great characteristic. Constant ineffectual urging to stool, and when the stool dose not occur it is incomplete and unsatisfactory, as if apart remained behind. Absence of desire for defecation contrary indicates Nux. Inflammatory symptoms or pain generally contraindicates. Carbo Veg has urging, but it is due to wind, while opium and Bryonia have no urging at all.

ALUMINA: Chief among remedies for constipation due to dryness of the intestinal tract stands Alumina. There is diminished peristaltic movement and complete inertia of the rectum, so that we have the symptom, soft stool expelled. There is little or no urging to stool. The stool may be hard or knotty like sheep dung, or may be soft. It is one of our most useful remedies in constipation of children where the rectum is dry, inflamed and bleeding about the orifice. Alumina differs from Bryonia chiefly in the state of rectal inactivity. A dry mouth and an irritated looking tongue may lead to the selection of Alumina. There is much straining with the remedy and the stool is passed in very small quantities. Constipation of infants and old people from inactive rectum, and in women of sedentary habit. Evacuation preceded by painful urging long before stool, and then straining at stool. Abnormal cravings- chalk, charcoal, dry food, tea grounds. Aversion to meat. No desire to eat.

BRYONIA: The large- hard dry stools as if burnt. The constipation is due to the dryness and there is no urging. The stools are passed with great difficulty, due to inactivity of the rectum. It cures the constipation, which is produced as a result of decreased intestinal secretions and decreased action of the muscular walls. In young children constipation is cured by the use of Bryonia. It acts better in summer and in rheumatic subjects. Stools brown, thick, bloody; worse in the morning, from moving, in hot weather, after being heated, from cold drinks. Thirst for large quantities of water at long intervals. Stomach sensitive to touch. Tongue coated yellowish dark brown, heavily white in gastric derangements. Vomiting of bile and water immediately after eating. Bryonia affects especially the constitution of a robust, firm fibre and dark complexion, with tendency to leanness and irritability. The Bryonia patient is irritable, has vertigo from raising the head. Feeling of a stone in the stomach.

OPIUM: The constipation of Opium is due to absolute inaction of the intestines, a regular paralysis of the peristaltic movement. There is an absence of desire, absolutely no urging to stool and so the faeces become impacted in the bowels; and when passed at all come in little, hard, dry, black balls like sheep dung. There is a want of sensibility throughout the intestinal tract, and consequently the constipation is not apt to inconvenience the patient, hence it is apt to go on getting worse until the attention is called to it by the flatus accumulating in the upper part of the intestines. When the faeces require artificial means for their removal, this remedy should be thought of. Diminished secretions are also a characteristic of Opium and dryness and intestinal inactivity is one of the causes of constipation in this remedy. It is indicated especially in constipation of old people, the patient is dull and dizzy. Violent pain in rectum. Abdomen is hard, bloated and tympanitic. During colic, urging to stool and discharge of hard faeces.

SULPHUR: There is an ineffectual urging to stool, with a sensation of heat and discomfort in the rectum, and there is uneasy feeling all through the intestinal tract, due to abdominal plethora or passive portal congestion. It is very useful remedy with which to commence the treatment of constipation. A bad constipation and frequent ill health are good indications for this remedy. The stools are hard, dark, dry and expelled with great straining the first effort to stool being extremely painful. There is apt to be much twitching and burning of the anus, the evacuations are often unsatisfactory and there is a sensation as if a part is left behind. Another characteristic of Sulphur is that diarrhoea alternates with constipation. Child is afraid to pass stools on account of pain. Redness around the anus, with itching. Complete loss of, or excessive appetite. Great desire for sweets. Drinks much, eat little. Milk disagrees. Very weak and faint at 11.am. must have something to eat.

❑❑❑

CHAPTER 17

Cough

This is the commonest symptom of nearly all respiratory diseases and is indicative of an effort to expel a foreign substance causing irritation on any place in the cough reflex path.

The center is in the medulla close to the respiratory centers. This is activated reflexly by the afferent impulses traveling up mostly along the vagus and to a less extent, the vagus and the phrenic (to bronchi and diaphragm), the spinal accessory, intercostals and other nerves supplying the accessory muscles of respiration. The peripheral fibres of the vagus and the phrenic are also sometimes directly affected causing cough reflex.

The medullary center itself may also be excited or restrained by impulses from superior cerebella centers, so that cough may be induced or controlled by voluntary efforts.

Cough Reflex

(a) *Vagus* : The exciting cause may be in the larynx, trachea, lungs, pleurae, oesophagus, stomach, intestine or other abdominal viscera.

Also in heart as in pulmonary congestion (cardiac branches), ear as in middle ear disease even wax in the ears (Arnold's branch to the ear) and the meninges.

(b) *Glosso-pharyngeal* : An irritating process may be present in the pharynx, tonsils and uvula.

(c) *Trigeminal* : The cough is occasionally of nasal origin may follow sneezing and sometimes result from a strong or pungent smell.

(d) *Phrenic :* Irritation of the diaphragm subphrenic or liver abscess, perinephritis may cause cough.

(e) *Psycogenic :* Sometimes especially in young females recurrent paroxysms of cough may be a psychogenic disturbances.

Thus, cough is usually due to disturbances in the respiratory passage or pleurae, irritation in the nose and the ear or sometimes in the abdominal viscera inflammation or irritation and occasionally cardiac decompensation.

It is important to make a note of the age of the patient, duration of the cough also what part of the day or night it is worst, voice is affected or not and if paroxysmal, painful or associated with any change of posture or vomiting.

In the morning cough is often due to bronchitis, bronchiectasis or tuberculous cavity. Night's accumulated secretion is coughed out.

Just on going to bed- enlarged uvula or laryngeal irritability.

On change of posture, the patient lying on the diseased side; pulmonary cavity or bronchiectasis (sputum trickles into the healthy bronchus), on the healthy side pleurisy or pneumonia.

Paroxysmal cough: whooping cough, laryngitis, chronic bronchitis, bronchiectasis and pressure of enlarged tracheo bronchial glands on the bronchi.

Suppressed cough is in a painful condition in the chest especially in pleurisy.

Cough with vomiting is in whooping cough or tonsillitis.

After exertion, congestive cardiac failure and on taking a meal, dyspepsia.

The Character of the Cough

If expectoration is absent non-productive cough, either there is simple congestion of the mucous membranes especially of the upper respiratory tract or such extra- pulmonary conditions as pleurisy or it is a reflex from other viscera.

If the expectoration productive coughs, exudates or transudates have collected in the bronchial passages, the sputum is thick in the distal bronchioles. As the sputum advances near to the larger bronchi by tissue squeeze, secretory pressure and respiratory movements, it is diluted and gets thinner.

Dry Cough

PHARYNX: Irritating hawking cough, persistent with little expectoration often followed by vomiting. If the uvula is enlarged, the cough is especially worse at night. Look for local signs in the pharynx as of pharyngitis or enlarged tonsils, adenoids and uvula.

NOSE: Chronic rhinitis especially with suppuration of the maxillary antrum, the cough may be in paroxysm.

LARYNX: Cough is often ineffectual and painful; the characteristic localizing sign is huskiness of the voice. In laryngitis the cough is noisy, husky, stridulus, paralysis of one of the vocal cords causes "brassy "cough and bilateral adductor paralysis " bovine" cough. In destructive lesion of the vocal cords, cough becomes toneless whispering.

TRACHEA: Brassy cough, often paroxysmal, usually due to pressure of an aneurysm, enlarged glands or of a tumour.

BRONCHIOLES AND LUNGS: Early stage of acute bronchitis, influenza, pulmonary tuberculosis and lobar pneumonia also whooping cough.

PLEURA: Short, painful suppressed cough.

STOMACH AND INTESTINE: Cough is sometimes associated with flatulent dyspepsia. Diarrhoea, constipation or intestinal helminthiasis and occasionally gastroduodenal ulcer and appendicitis may cause cough.

EAR: Impacted wax, frunculosis, eczema and mechanical irritation of the external auditory meatus excite cough.

PERICARDITIS: Dry nonproductive cough may be present.

The character of the sputum is of great diagnostic value.

Lobar pneumonia: Expectoration is at first scanty, sticky and rusty afterwards at the stage of resolution, more copious, greenish, yellow or white.

Bronchitis: in acute stage, the sputum is scanty, thin and frothy, in a chronic case, copious mucopurulent even foetid.

Bronchiectasis, pulmonary cavity: paroxysmal cough especially in the morning with copious foetid expectoration usually excited or aggravated by change of posture.

Lung abscess or gangrene: foetid sputum with lung debris.

Rupture into a bronchus of empyema or liver abscess the appearance of the pus is characteristic.

Homoeopathic Medicines

BRYONIA: There is dry cough in the Bryonia. It seems to come from the stomach, and is preceded by a tickling in the epigastrium. During the cough the patient holds the sides of the chest with his hands, as the cough not only shakes the chest, but also hurts distant parts of the body. It is aggravated by coming from the open air into a warm room and is accompanied by bursting headache. The expectoration is scanty, tough and sometimes bloody. The cough of Bryonia is looser and more moist than that of Aconite, and there are usually sharp stitching pleuritic pains, the cough of Bryonia is also hard and dry at times and the sputum is scanty and rust coloured. There may be circumscribed redness of the cheeks, slight delirium and apathy, the tongue will most likely to be dry, and the patient will want to keep perfectly quiet. It is right-sided remedy and attacks the parenchyma of the lung, and is perhaps more strongly indicated in the croupous form of pneumonia.

PHOSPHORUS: The cough of Phosphorus arises from irritation in the trachea. The patient is worse by talking or using the voice; any change in breathing causes cough. It is at first dry and tight and then with expectoration of tenacious purulent mucus. It is worse from a change to cold air, the chest feels dry and the cough sounds dry, and there is a constriction across the upper part of the chest. Continued hoarseness with a distressing dry cough. Congestion of lungs sharp stitches in chest respiration quickened oppressed tuberculosis in tall, rapidly growing young people. There is cough, with pain under sternum, as if something were torn loose; there is pressure across the upper part of the chest and constriction of the larynx; there are mucous rales; labored breathing, sputa yellowish mucus, with blood streaks therein, or rust colored, as under Bryonia.

RUMEX CRISPUS: This remedy has a dry cough from tickling in the supra-sternal fossa. It is laryngo tracheal cough, which is teasing and persistent, and is aggravated by cold air. The patient has to cover the head with the bedclothes and breathe warm air to stop the cough. Deep inspiration aggravates the cough. It suits incessant fatiguing cough, with soreness behind the sternum, and much tough mucus in the larynx, which cannot be hawked up. It suits the night coughs of consumptive where there are sharp, stitching pains through the lungs in the early stages.

ANTIMONIUM TART: The cough is loose and the patient feels sure that the next cough will raise the mucus; but it does not, no phlegm is raised. There is drowsiness accompanying the cough and the dsypnoea increases. There is rattling in the chest and the absence of expectoration. It is a convulsive, concussive cough, attended with copious secretion of mucus. It is worse at night and in bed. The expectoration when present is either lemon yellow or blood streaked. With Antimonium tart there is great oppression of breathing, worse towards morning, compelling the patient to sit up to breathe. There are also sharp, stitching pains and high fever, perhaps it corresponds more to the catarrhal form than it does to the croupous form. Oedema and impending paralysis of lungs. Bronchial tubes loaded with mucus. Cough excited by eating, with pain in chest and larynx. Dizziness with cough. Dsypnoea relieved by eructation. Cough and dyspnoea better by lying on right side.

□□□

CHAPTER 18

Dandruff

The term dandruff includes several different conditions of the scalp. There is scaling in which the entire scalp may be covered with loose dry scales. When the hair is combed or brushed, or when the scalp is scratched, these scales fall like snow on the shoulders. Often there is itching, as well, and the scalp may be red from scratching.

What is at first thought to be dandruff may later prove to be some other conditions, such as *seborrhoeic dermatitis,* or worse still *psoriasis* and even *neurodermatitis.*

Neurodermatitis : It is a chronic type of itching and inflammation of the skin. The itching area may be in some localized spot or it may extend over large areas of the body. The condition may even develop in infants. It may disappear after the age of two and return in the early teens of later. The condition is more often seen in those who suffer from fever, hives and asthma. True cause is not known for most of the people are allergic to many things. Many of them are tense and restless and are troubled with a dry skin. They are hypersensitive and are often given to itching, especially in the bend of elbow or behind the knee. The constant scratching leaves deep scratch marks and causes thickening and furrowing of the skin.

Seborrhoeic dermatitis : It is a chronic inflammation of the skin most frequently seen on the scalp. The true cause is not known. Inflammation may begin on the skin behind the ears. Later the whole scalp may be involved including the external ear canals. From there it may spread to the eyebrows, the folds of the nose, and the front of the chest. Reddish, scaling patches may also appear under the breasts and in the body creases, especially around the groin and anal areas.

If the scalp is covered with greasy scales, wash the hair thoroughly every day, using some good soap or medicated shampoo. Frequent washing will not harm the hair.

Itching lesions of the scalp are often due to *neurodermatitis* especially when it occurs on the back of the head.

Keep the hair and scalp clean by frequent shampoo. Clean your comb and brush after each use. Follow the directions suggested for more stubborn cases of dandruff, and do not scratch.

A number of lotions are available in the market for skin diseases. But they only suppress the disease to bring more severe cases. True treatment lies in homoeopathy. There is a very good treatment for dandruff in homoeopathy, which is given as under:

Homoeopathic Medicines

ARSENIC ALB: It irritates, inflames, and destroys all tissues. It acts rapidly and violently. Burning is the ranking sensation. A useful remedy in all cases of skin troubles when the skin is thickened. The sensations are itching, burning and swelling, it also has papules, nettle rash and pimples. Burning sensitive ulcers with offensive discharges. It is perhaps our best general remedy for the chronic form of eczema with great burning and itching. It is almost a specific for hives from fish, which burn and for repercussed hives pustules form into scabs. Itching, burning, swellings; oedema, eruption, popular, dry, rough, scaly, worse cold and scratching. Malignant pustules. Ulcers with offensive discharge. Urticaria with burning and restlessness. Icy coldness of body. Gangrenous inflammation. Scalp itches intolerable; circular patches of bare spots, rough, dirty, sensitive and covered with dry scales; nightly burning and itching; dandruff. Scalp very sensitive cannot brush hair.

GRAPHITES: Sensation of cobweb on forehead. Burning on vertex. Humid, itching eruption on hairy scalp, emitting a fetid odor. The sensations are itching, burning and swelling, it also has papules, nettle rash and pimples. Burning sensitive ulcers with offensive discharges. It is perhaps our best general remedy for the chronic form of eczema with great burning and itching. It is almost a specific for hives from fish, which burn and for repercussed hives pustules form into scabs. Itching, burning, swellings; oedema, eruption, popular, dry, rough, scaly, worse cold and scratching. Malignant pustules. Ulcers with offensive discharge. Urticaria with burning and restlessness. Icy coldness of body. Gangrenous inflammation. Moisture and eruption behind the ears. Fissures in and behind the ear. Thin, white, scaly membrane covering membrane tympani.

THUJA: White, scaly dandruff; hair dry and falling out. Greasy skin of face. Pain in the head as if pierced by nail. Acts on skin, blood, gastrointestinal tract, kidneys and brain. Its relation to the production of pathological vegetations condylomate, warty excrescences spongy tumors is very important. Dry skin with brown spots. Eruptions only on covered parts; worse after scratching. Very sensitive to touch. Freckles and blotches. Perspiration sweetish and strong.

NATRUM MUR: A great remedy for certain forms of intermittent fever, anaemia, chlorosis, many disturbances of the alimentary tract and skin. Dry mucous membrane. Oversensitive to all sorts of influences. Skin greasy, oily especially on hairy parts. Dry eruptions especially on margins of hairy scalp and bends of joints. Urticaria itch and burn. Crusty eruptions in bends of limbs, margin of scalp, behind ears. Eczema raw, red and inflamed, worse eating salt at seashore. Affects hair follicles. Hives itching after exertion. Face is oily as if greased. Earthy complexion of the face. Patient is irritable and gets into a passion about trifles. Wants to be alone to cry. Tears with laughter. Great weariness and weakness. Anaemic headache of school girls. Chronic headache, semi lateral, congestive, from sunrise to sunset, with pale face, nausea and vomiting.

SEPIA: Herpes behind ears on nape of neck. Pain as if from sub-cutaneous ulceration. Swelling and eruption of external ear. Yellow blotches on face. Hair falls out. Coldness of vertex. Pimples on forehead near hair. Herpes circinatus in isolated spots. Itching not relieved by scratching; worse in bends of elbows and knees. Herpetic eruption on lips, about mouth and nose. Urticaria on going in open air; better in warm room. Itching with offensive odor of skin.

□□□

CHAPTER 19

Depression

Individuals suffering from the more pronounced types of mental disorder are sometimes said to be insane, but the term insanity is a legal one, not a medical term. An insane person is one who cannot distinguish right from wrong or assume responsibilities for his own actions. In the case of a psychotic patient the whole personality is involved. And he is completely out of touch with real world around. Not so the neurotic patient. Only a small part of his personality is involved. Psychotic patients often require hospitalization; neurotic patients rarely do, unless they have some additional physical problem.

Another distinction between these two major groups is that his friends usually bring the psychotic patient to the doctor, while the neurotic comes of his own accord. He knows he is sick, and he usually wants help. Most often he is suffering from a nervous depression.

Reactive depression: This is a simple depression or sadness which is usually brought on by some catastrophe or unhappy event, such as losing one's home or business in a fire, or perhaps by the death of some loved one in the family. When something like this happens most people passed through a few days or weeks of sadness and then try to carry on as best they can. The patient with a reactive depression seems unable to do this. His grief lasts a long time, and he may be so disturbed as to be unable to do his normal work.

Why is he now so deeply depressed? A careful survey of his early childhood will probably show some real problems. And while such a person may have appeared to be perfectly normal all his life there may have been times when he felt his whole world was more or less falling apart. In spite of this he was able to get along somehow but he always felt somewhat weakened and deprived of the normal satisfactions of life. The recent catastrophe such as losing his business may have been more than he could take— — the last straw.

Physiotherapy or mind treatment is advisable in all cases of reactive depression. It is most important for the patient to gain an insight into why he is so depressed. This will help to prevent further episodes. If he becomes so severely depressed as to contemplate suicide, he should be given a series of electric shock treatments to help him over his depression.

Delayed Grief Reaction. When some loved one dies, it is perfectly natural to weep. Failure to grieve may indicate some personality disturbance that should be corrected. These peculiar mixed or ambivalent feelings are often a sign that all is not well. A normal amount of grief is nature's way of releasing tensions. Abnormal reactions should be discussed with someone who understands the mechanism of the human mind, so that a more normal response will develop. This may help to avert a complete mental breakdown in future.

Attempted suicide. Some people threaten to commit suicide mainly to see how the family will react. They may never actually carry this out, but such threats should always be taken seriously, for they indicate a troubled mind. Also the time may come when they may become depressed enough to carry it out. Remember, the person who never smiles is always depressed. Strangely, the greatest risk is when he appears taking a turn for the better. This may be the moment when he plans to end his life.

The homoeopathic treatment for a depressed patient is given as under:

Homoeopathy Medicines

BELLADONNA: It is one of the important remedies for delirious states, and must be given where there is wildness, restlessness and a desire to cut or tear the clothing. The patient springs out of bed and strikes those around him. He appears frightened and sees objects when he closes his eyes. Speech and actions are hasty. Violence is great characteristic, great noisiness, the patient sings, screams and curses. Belladonna patent is extremely depressed, fearful and subject to violent attacks of weeping. Patient lives in a world of his own. Hallucinations; sees monsters, hideous faces. Delirium, frightful images. Loss of consciousness. Disinclined to talk. Acuteness of all senses.

ARSENIC ALB: Useful for the depressed delirious, fear of death, fear of being alone, with strong suicidal tendencies. See ghosts and vermin, crawling on bed. It relieves the tendency in the insane to the mutilation of the body, pricking at the skin until it sore; chewing finger nails etc. exhaustive insanity and acute delirious mania with typhoid symptoms and rapid exhaustion, acute melancholia. Restlessness, thirst, physical exhaustion and midnight aggravation. Thinks it is useless to take medicine. Suicidal tendencies. Sensitive to disorder and confusion.

NATRUM MUR: The patient requiring this remedy is melancholic, hypochondriac, sad and hopeless about the future, easily angered, Patients shed floods of tears, consolation aggravates. There is emaciation and prematurely aged look. There is a persistent recalling of past unpleasant experiences and grievances. His memory is poor, conversation disconnected, has hallucinations of hearing and delusions. Ill effects of grief, fright, anger etc. depressed particularly in chronic diseases. Irritable gets into a passion about trifles. Wants to be alone to cry. Tears with laughter.

PULSATILLA: The disposition and mental state are the chief guiding symptoms of this remedy. It is especially suited to mild, gentle, yielding females. Sad, crying readily; weeps when talking. The patient seeks the open air; always feel better there, even though the patient is chilly. Patient is timid and irresolute. Fears in evening to be alone. Likes sympathy. Easily discouraged. Highly emotional. Given to extremes of pleasure and pain. Morbid dread of the opposite sex.

IGNATIA: Produces a marked hyperasthesia of all the senses and a tendency to clonic spasms. It is one of the chief remedies for hysteria. It is especially adapted to the nervous temperament, women of sensitive nature, easily excited, and dark, mild disposition. Rapid change of physical and mental conditions, opposite to each other. Alert, nervous, apprehensive, rigid, trembling patients who suffer acutely in mind and body, a t the same time made worse by drinking coffee. Effects of grief and worry. Changeable mood; silently brooding. Melancholic, sad and tearful. Not communicative. Sighing and sobbing. It is indicated after shocks, grief, and disappointment. The patient hides her grief, is introspective, changeable and silent. It is a remedy full of jealousy and disappointments. The patient refuses sympathy. The patient has a disposition to brood over her sorrows.

CIMICIFUGA: In depressed states this is one of our best remedies. The patient is weak, depressed, "shrouded in a dark, heavy, mental atmosphere"; Suspicious people and objects appear strange and unnatural, the brain feels too large. There is a sensation of pall of gloom or horrible sadness, settling over her mind is the great characteristic of the remedy. It is expressed as a feeling as if something is going to happen, or as if they were going crazy. It thus becomes a suitable remedy in melancholia and in puerperal mania.

Visions of rats and mice are sometimes seen and the remedy has been successfully used in delirium tremens.

ANACARDIUM: A most valuable remedy in mental states and its most important characteristics is the sensation of having two wills, one urging him to do and other forbids. Another characteristic is the patient's irritability, with an irresistible desire to swear and curse. Anacardium also has loss of memory. The patient will imagine that he hears voices a far off talking to him, or he has a fixed idea that he is possessed of a devil, that he is double, or a women will think that her child is not her own. It is indicated in low melancholic conditions. In chronic mania it is more often curative than any other remedy.

CHAPTER 20

Eczema

Eczema is a troublesome skin condition characterized by redness, cracking, oozing and scaling of the skin. Extremes of heat and cold and even emotional stress seem to play a part in this condition. The patient usually complains of itching and burning in the skin, especially at the night. Sores appear on various parts of the body, but most often on the hands, feet, ears and legs. Eczema may come on at any time of life and in either sex. The commoner manifestations are erythema changing to papule, vesicle, crust, scale and fissure, with serous exudation. In chronic cases, thick scales accumulate.

This is the effect of local irritation by chemical, thermal, actinic or mechanical agents in a hypersensitive individual, subject of an allergy or constitutional disabilities such as gout, chronic nephritis, rheumatism, local sepsis, dyspepsia, alcoholism, uterine disturbances also teething. In some cases heredity may be found.

Papules, vesicles and pustules with some degree of local oedema are found; exudation, crusting and scaling with inflammation of varying severity may be present. These tend to spread to the contiguous areas.

One or both cheeks of an infant or the ear, limbs or trunk are occasionally involved. In adults also similar papulo- vesicular eruptions appear. Sensations of burning, smarting, throbbing or itching are present, according to the acuteness of the process and severity of the inflammation.

When chronic the discharge diminishes or disappears, leaving a thickened, irregular, scaly patch, fading at the margins.

In homoeopathy there is a very good treatment for every skin disease, so is for eczema. The following medicines are useful in cases of eczema:

Homoeopathic Medicines

RHUS TOX: Vesicular eruptions are a characteristic of this remedy. It is useful in herpes, eczema, pemphigus and prurigo. It is useful in right-sided zoster with extensive vesication and perhaps accompanied with rheumatic pains. The skin is covered with numerous vesicles, there is great itching and tingling, the skin is often swollen and oedematous and these vesicles have a red areola around them. The symptoms are all worse at night, in damp weather and in winter. Rapid vesication and red eruptions on the skin. Glands swollen. Burning eczematous eruptions with tendency to scale formation. Ailments from strains, over lifting, while perspiring. Septic conditions. Cellulites and infections, carbuncles in early stages.

PSORINUM: Herpetic eruptions with much itching, worse when getting warm in bed, the skin is dirty, greasy, unwashed in appearance. Tinea capitis, offensive matter oozes out. Sebaceous glands secrete in excess. Eczema more on the sides of head and face, cheeks and ears. Eruption in the bends of joints. Pustules or boils remaining after itch. A most important remedy in all skin affections. Skin is dirty and dingy looking. Dry, lusterless, rough hair. Intolerable itching. Indolent ulcers slow to heal. Crusty eruptions all over. Pustules near finger nails. Urticaria after every exertion. Easy perspiration when walking. Offensive discharges. Extreme sensitiveness to cold, wants the head warm, wants warm clothing even in summer.

GRAPHITES: The corners of the mouth and eyes are cracked, bleeding and oozing a gluey, thick, tenacious discharge, a fissured eczema is the type. Great itching is always accompanying the eruption. The skin may be dry and horny. The hair is dry and falls out. Rough, hard, persistent dryness of portions of skin unaffected by eczema. Eruption oozing out a sticky exudation. Our great remedy for all sorts of skin diseases. The symptoms calling for it are very clear; there are moist scabby eruptions on the scalp, face, and bends of joints, between fingers and behind the ears. Every little injury suppurates. Cracks in nipples, mouth, between toes, anus. Burning and stinging pain. Ulcers discharging a glutinous fluid, thin and sticky. Pimples and acne.

ARSENIC ALB: It irritates, inflames, and destroys all tissues. It acts rapidly and violently. Burning is the ranking sensation. A useful remedy in all cases of skin troubles when the skin is thickened, such as in chronic eczema, psoriasis and chronic urticaria. The sensations are itching, burning and swelling, it also has papules, nettle rash and pimples. Burning sensitive ulcers with offensive discharges. It is perhaps our best general remedy for the chronic form of eczema with great burning and itching. It is almost a specific for hives from fish, which burn and for repercussed hives pustules form into scabs. Itching, burning, swellings; oedema, eruption, popular, dry, rough, scaly, worse cold and scratching. Malignant pustules. Ulcers with offensive discharge. Urticaria with burning and restlessness. Icy coldness of body. Gangrenous inflammation.

SULPHUR: The great characteristic of this remedy is the aggravation from washing; this with scratching makes the parts burn intensely. The skin is rough, coarse and measly, and there is much soreness in the fold of the skin and a tendency to pustular eruptions. Dryness and heat of scalp, with intense itching, especially at night and scratching causes soreness; wetting makes it burn. Eczema erthematosum. Eruption of yellow crusts. Eruptions at the margin of the hair. Dry, scaly, unhealthy; every little injury suppurates. Itching, burning, worse scratching and washing. Excoriation especially in folds. Feeling of a band around bones. Skin affections after local medication. Purities especially from warmth, in evening, often occur in springtime, in damp weather.

HEPAR SULPHURIS: Moist eruption in folds of skin and itching in the bends of joints; the skin is extremely sensitive and suppurates easily, and pimples form around ulcers. Humid eczema of the scalp, sore and sensitive to touch. Eczema of the scrotum and genital organs boils. It is especially useful after the abuse of intents containing zinc and mercury. Suppurative glands are very sensitive. Papules prone to suppurate and extend. Acne in youth. Suppurate with pricky pain. Easily bleed. Angio-neurotic oedema. Unhealthy skin; every little injury suppurates. Chapped skin, with deep cracks on hands and feet. Ulcers with bloody suppuration. Smelling like old cheese. Ulcers very sensitive to contact, burning, stinging, and easily bleeding. Sweats day and night without relief. " Cold sores" very sensitive. Cannot bear to be uncovered; wants to be wrapped up warmly. Sticking or pricking in afflicted parts. Putrid ulcers, surrounded by little pimples. Great sensitiveness to slightest touch. Chronic and recurring urticaria. Small pox, herpes circinatus. Constant offensive exhalation from the body.

SILICIA: Felons, abscesses, boils, and old fistulous ulcers. Delicate, pale, waxy. Cracks at end of fingers. Painless swelling of glands. Rose coloured blotches. Scars suddenly become painful. Pus offensive. Promotes expulsion of foreign bodies from tissues. Every long lasting suppuration and fistulous tracts. Dry fingertips. Eruptions itch only in daytime and evening. Crippled nails. Indurated tumors. Abscesses of joints. After impure vaccination. Nodes and coppery spots. Keloid growths.

CHAPTER 21

Gallstones

The gall bladder is a small, pear shaped, muscular organ closely attached to the under surface of the liver. Its only function is to store and concentrate the bile between meals so there will be a plentiful supply when needed. Bile from the liver is a clear, golden colour when formed, but after being concentrated in the gall bladder it turns a deep green. This concentrating process sometimes results in the formation of stones in the gall bladder, particularly following pregnancy in commonly over weight women. Many people with gallstones seem to have no problem at all, especially if there is one large stone. But when a number of smaller stones are present in the gall bladder, the patient may feel sharp, cramp like pains all over the upper abdomen.

The predisposing causes are stagnation of bile, due to an excessive diet of starch and fat, constipation, obesity, pregnancy, tight lacing or other obstruction to the flow of bile.

The exciting causes are catarrhal and infective inflammation of the gall bladder, like sepsis, typhoid etc., and tumors. Old patients and women are most susceptible.

The symptoms vary as much as do the consistency and shape of the stones. In the acute form (hepatic colic), we have cutting, burning, tearing, lancinating pains in the right hypochondriac region extending to the shoulder. The pains begin at a point two and a half inches to the right of the median line and the same distance below the ensiform cartilage. Occasionally, the seat of the pain is in the immediate region of the gall bladder. Chills often precede an attack; nausea and vomiting; profuse cold sweat; feeble rapid pulse; jaundice. In a majority of cases, there is a slight elevation in the region of the liver felt below the margin of the ribs sometimes as low as the umbilical line; also tenderness between the tenth and twelfth ribs at the right of the spine which is a ranking symptom.

We should also remember that hepatic calculi of considerable size are often found in the feces which have produced no symptoms whatever; that there may be recurrences of the attacks (frequently at the time of the menses), or that the stones being expelled, the attack cease to return. The duration of an attack varies from a few hours to a few weeks.

Gallstones are sometimes mistaken for gastralgia. In the latter we have the neurotic history, the history of the attacks, amelioration from firm pressure over the epigastria and absence of fever, jaundice and stones in the stools; also amelioration. From food, will easily determine.

Renal colic, in which the pain begins over the kidney bladder of the affected side, runs down the ureter to the bladder; in which there is also pain and retraction of the testicle; and a scanty, irregular amount of the urine which is often mixed with blood.

Enteralgia, in which the pains are more of a twisting, boring, squeezing nature, usually amelioration by pressure or the passing of flatus.

Reflex colic, especially when due to ovarian and uterine troubles, is more difficult to differentiate. In many cases the diagnosis cannot be made without entering the abdomen.

Chronic obstruction of the gall ducts; cholangitis varies from biliary calculi in a few particulars both as to its symptomology and pathology. The cholangitis may be either simple or suppurative. In the simple form, the gall bladder is somewhat enlarged; the common duct is greatly distended; the hepatic duct and its branches are not only distended and their lining membrane smooth and clear, but they often contain a thin, colourless mucus. The mucous membrane is greatly swollen and reddened in suppurative cholangitis, and may have erosions and even ulcers. Infection of the liver and formation of abscesses may include other organs.

From the above, we see that many symptoms may be added to those of the non-obstructive form. They are jaundice, constant or intermittent; temprature at first paroxysmal, later remittent or even intermittent; and also the symptoms of strictures, fistula, adhesions, etc.

Homoeopathic Medicines

Chelidonium : Jaundice due to hepatic and gall bladder obstruction. Gall colic. Distention. Fermentation and sluggish bowels. Liver enlarged. Gall stones. Urine profuse, foaming, yellow urine, like beer. Dark and turbid. Tongue yellow with imprint of teeth, large and flabby. Prefers hot food and drink. Pain through stomach to back and right shoulder blade. Gastralgia. Eating relieves temporarily, especially when accompanied with hepatic symptoms. Stools hard, round balls like sheep's dung, bright yellow, stools float in water.

Lycopodium : Pain shooting across lower abdomen from right to left. Dropsy due to hepatic disease. Immediately after eating a light meal, abdomen is bloated, full. Liver sensitive. Brown spots on abdomen. Stools hard, difficult, small, and incomplete. Pain in back before urinating; ceases after flow; slow in coming, must strain. Retention. Polyuria during the night. Heavy red sediment. Desire for sweet things. Aversion to bread, etc. after eating pressure in stomach, with bitter taste in mouth. Eating ever so little creates fullness.

Nux vomica : Bruised soreness of abdominal walls. Flatulent distention with spasmodic colic. Liver engorged with stitches and soreness. Colic with upward pressure, causing short breathe, and desire for stool. Weakness of abdominal ring region. Forcing in lower abdomen towards genitals. Constipation with frequent ineffectual urging, incomplete and unsatisfactory; feeling as if part remained unexpelled. Alternate constipation and diarrhoea-after abuse of purgatives. Scanty stool, with much urging. Renal colic extending to genitals, with dribbling urine. While urinating, itching in urethra and pain in neck of bladder. Haematuria. Ineffectual urging, spasmodic and strangury.

Chionanthus : Hepatic derangements, jaundice, enlarged spleen. It is a prominent liver remedy. Aching in umbilical region, griping. Feels as if strings were tied in a "slip- knot" around intestines, which was suddenly drawn tight and then gradually loosened. Sore, enlarged, with jaundice and constipation. Clay-cloured stool also soft, yellow and pasty. Tongue heavily coated. No appetite. Bilious colic. Hepatic region tender. There is large amount of high specific gravity in the urine, frequent urination, bile and sugar in the urine, urine very dark.

Calcarea carb : Gall stone colic. Increase of fat in abdomen. Cannot bear tight clothing around the waist. Distension with hardness. Cutting in abdomen. Swollen abdomen. Sensitive to slightest pressure. Liver region painful when stooping. Stool large and hard whitish, watery. Diarrhoea of undigested food, fetid with ravenous appetite. Constipation; stool at first hard, then pasty, then liquid. Urine dark, brown, sour, fetid, abundant with white sediment, bloody.

Belladonna : Cutting pain across; stitches in left side of abdomen, when coughing, sneezing or touching it. Extreme sensitiveness to touch, bedclothes, etc. abdomen is distended and hot. Pain as if clutched by a hand; worse jars; pressure. Spasmodic pain in epigastrium. Constriction pain runs to spine. Nausea and vomiting. Great thirst for cold water. Spasms of stomach. Dread of drinking. Stools thin, green, and dysenteric, in lumps like chalk. Shuddering during stool. Acute urinary infections. Sensation of motion in bladder as of a worm. Urine scanty, with tenesmus; dark and turbid, loaded with phosphates. Urine frequent and profuse. Haematuria where no pathological condition can be found.

❑❑❑

CHAPTER 22

Gastric Ulcer

Gastric Ulcer a well defined ulcer involving the mucous membrane of the stomach with a tendency to progressive destruction, beginning in the mucosa and sometimes extending to and even through the deeper layers of the walls of the stomach.

We have not been able to name a definite cause. "Altered composition of the blood and the resulting insufficient nourishment of the cells". Riegel says the ulcer is due "to a self-digestion of the stomach at the limited spot." He calls attention to the fact that the gastric juice is always hyperacid in these cases and thinks it is more than a mere coincidence. Virchow says the cause is emboli or thrombi, which form in the nutrient gastric arteries, which have lost their tonicity. He claims that an ulcer forms at the point of obstruction.

Gastric ulcers occur most frequently between twenty and thirty years of age. This is an average, which we arrive at from the fact that in females it is from fifteen to thirty and in males from forty to forty-five. The predominance of women over men as shown by clinical statistics is two to one, but pathologically the numbers are about equal in two sexes.

No occupation seems to grant exemption. Cooks seems to be more predisposed. Next come metal workers in those factories where there is much dust. Some claim that shoemakers and tailors are also prone to the condition.

The trauma may be external or internal. Internal trauma may result from hot foods or drinks, foreign bodies, corrosives, mechanical and chemical irritants. These results, however, differ in their pathology as well as their course from the regular gastric ulcer.

Anemia, chlorosis and menstrual disorders are frequently predisposing causes. I feel confident that gastric ulcers, which are found in patients suffering from dysentery, syphilis and tuberculosis, differ from the genuine gastric ulcer, which we are discussing.

The location of these ulcers may be wherever the gastric juice is found. The posterior surface of the stomach is the most common site, 42 percent of all cases are found there, especially near the pylorus and along the lower curvature. Gastric ulcers are usually single, occasionally multiple. When multiple they may be of the same duration, but as rule some are in the state of healing, while others seem to be of recent origin.

The more acute ulcers have a punched, sharp appearance, round or oval and sharp in outline. Ulcers in the later stage vary somewhat from the acute, being self-shaped, i.e., the widest diameter being at the mucosa. The usual size varies from two to four cm. and again some have been found whose diameter was 10 cm.

Microscopic examination shows the tissues to be necrotic. There is very little inflammation about the acute gastric ulcer, which in a measure accounts for the slow repair and healing.

Healing and cicatrisation are common. There is no doubt that we have many superficial types of erosion, which never become real ulcers, which heal with granulation from the submucosa and leave scar tissue.

Perforation takes place when the ulcer penetrates down to the serosa before adhesions have formed, and for this reason it naturally occurs most commonly on the anterior wall.

The symptoms are pain, tenderness, vomiting, and hemorrhage from the stomach. The sensations are gnawing, burning, sticking and sharp. The modalities are worse after eating; the agg. from pressure. There is amelioration after the stomach is empty, whether the emptiness is due to vomiting or the food passing out. Vomiting occurs after taking food and aggravates, if the food were highly seasoned, contains barriers or fibres. The hemorrhage also comes after eating. If soon after, the blood is bright red and pure; later it is darker and still later it may be almost black, the coffee grounds. The last shows the presence and action of the gastric juice upon the blood.

The pain, vomiting and hemorrhages are all aggravated by exertion, both physical and mental, especially emotions like fear and anger. Of the three conditions, pain is the most frequent vomiting, second in frequency, but hemorrhage out ranks them both in clinical important. Haemetamesis means ulceration in the great majority of cases, but the ulcers which given rise to it is not always gastric ulcers. Some times the blood from the ulcer passes through he intestines, causing a black tar like stool if the amount of blood were large. The hemorrhage from the duodenal ulcer passes through the intestines except that portion of blood, which is absorbed, by the elementary tract.

Homoeopathic Medicines

ARGENTUM NITRICUM : It has an elective affinity for the mucous membrane and submucosa and that its most frequent action is ulceration. The sensations are gripping with burning; gnawing; stinging ulcerative aggravated by touch and deep inspiration; burning; twisting and soreness. The pains extend from the stomach to the back, chest, shoulders, and down the abdomen. There is also a painful swelling of the pit of the stomach; stomach distended by gas with frequent eructation's. In addition to the above nausea, wretching and vomiting is also present. The vomited material staining the cloth black. With the vomiting, which is sometimes mucous, we often find a green mucous stool and occasionally, bloody stools. Complaints are aggravated from pressure, from deep inspiration, from eating or drinking and better by eructating gas, from vomiting.

ARSENIC ALB: It irritates, inflames, and destroys all tissues. It acts rapidly and violently. Burning is the ranking sensation. Eating and drinking, especially anything cold aggravates the pain and cause vomiting; rapid emaciation results from in ability of retaining the food. The stools are usually liquid and dark, often containing blood. The Arsenic patient is always fearful of the outcome of his condition. Great thirst drinks much but little at a time. Nausea, retching, vomiting after eating or drinking anxiety in pit of stomach. Vomiting of blood, bile, green mucous, or brown black mixed with blood. Gastralgia from slightest food or drink. Dyspepsia from vinegar, acids, ice cream and tobacco. Ill effects of vegetable diet, melons and watery fruits generally.

LACHESIS :It destroys the coagulating properties of the blood. It causes a tendency of all abscesses to become gangrenous. The Lachesis patient is dark with dark eyes, skin and hair of a nervous temperament. The most important symptom of this remedy is intolerance of anything tight about the stomach or abdomen. Gnawing and sticking pains are also present. The vomiting is usually of black blood. The abdomen is greatly distended, causing distress, aggravated by pressure of any kind. The stools are liquid and offensive, often dark containing blood. The excessive use of alcohol by the patient is an added indication for Lachesis. Empty swallowing more painful than swallowing salads. The aggravations are from sleep, hot weather, and from pressure of tight bandaging.

PHOSPHORUS: Inflammation of the stomach, with burning extending to throat and bowels. Bad effects of eating too much salt. Pain in stomach relieved by cold food. Region of stomach painful to touch or on walking. Belching large quantities of wind after eating. Vomiting water as soon as it gets warm in the stomach. Hunger soon after eating.

Sour taste and sour eructation after every meal. A very weak, empty gone sensation felt in the whole abdomen cavity. Very foetid stools and flatus. Great weakness after stool. Discharge of blood from rectum, during stool.

KALI BICHROMICUM: Round ulcer of stomach chronic intestinal ulceration cutting pain in abdomen soon after eating. Gastric symptoms are relieved after eating, and the rheumatic symptoms reappear. Vomiting of bright yellow water. Dilatation of stomach. Nausea and vomiting after beer. Load immediately after eating. Stools jelly like, gelatinous worse morning. Dislikes water cannot digest meat. Desire for beer and acids.

□□□

CHAPTER 23

Gastritis

Inflammation of the mucous membrane of the stomach, sometimes accompanied by more or less severe constitutional manifestations.

The predisposing causes are:

(1) The diatheses, especially those that affect the mucous membrane, tuberculous and cancerous, gouty and rheumatic.

(2) The various forms of anemia.

(3) Malnutrition.

(4) Chronic diseases, not only of the stomach but also of the other organs.

(5) Convalescence from acute diseases.

The exciting causes are:

(1) Diet, such as improper food; too hot or too cold food or drink; spoiled or too highly seasoned foods, canned goods and spoiled meats. To be a little more explicit. The ptomaines will produce gastric fever with typhoid and septic symptoms.

(2) Drugs including the gases.

(3) Infectious diseases.

(4) Animal parasites.

There are four stages of the disease: simple Acute, Chronic, Ulcerative and Suppurative.

The mind forms, as seen through gastric fistulae, present the following: Red, dry, ecchymosed spots; serum mixed with an increased mucus, escaped leucocytes, desquamated epithelium; erosions which bleed; later the mucous membrane becomes swollen, softened and covered with mucus and pus; the solitary lymph follicle swollen and infiltrated; small abscesses form, rupture and become ulcers; the gastric tubules filled with dead epithelium cells. Necrosis of the coats with sloughing and perforation may follow in the cases in which drugs are the cause.

Uneasiness, distress, distension, and pain is dull, sharp, burning, drawing, pulsating, and sticking in character. Nausea and vomiting is also present. Vomiting is sour, bitter or sweet. The vomiting may contain food in all degrees of digestion, in the toxic form, poison may be found in the vomit, shreds of mucous membrane, blood and pus. The tongue may be clean or coated. In the toxic form not only the tongue but the whole mucous membrane of the mouth may be discolored. In the chronic variety, the wall of the stomach may be thickened. There is a feeling of fullness in the abdomen. Prolonged illness results in loss of weight. In a few cases a small ulcer may be present which is not seen on X- ray. People with pernicious anaemia may suffer from atrophic gastritis due to loss of the "intrinsic" factor, which is normally present in the gastric juice.

The acute form is easily diagnosed by the vomiting which gives relief; temperature with sudden rise and sudden fall; pain and tenderness.

The chronic form by the fact that poison has been taken. An inspection of the mouth and pharynx will help; in other cases, a chemical examination of the stomach contents, the vomit and even the urine will be necessary.

In the acute, suppurative form a positive diagnosis is more difficult to make, especially in the diffuse variety, but the pus cells assist. A gastric abscess however is more easily diagnosed by the history of the case and the presence of a fluctuating tremor.

Homoeopathic Medicines

NUX VOMICA: The food and drink taste normal, and the gastric and abdominal disturbances do not begin immediately after eating. There is often nausea, empty retching, scanty, sour or bilious vomiting, water brash, sour, bitter, metallic or putrid taste, and vertigo is also present. All the symptoms are aggravated in the morning and also after eating dinner. The eructations are bitter, painful or sour. The nausea is especially after the meal. The stomach is sensitive to pressure and to tight clothing, and the patient will say: "If I could only vomit I would feel better." Important causes of dyspepsia are mental overwork, sedentary habits, high living and dissipation. Bruised soreness of abdominal walls. Flatulent distention with spasmodic colic. Liver engorged with stitches and soreness. Colic with upward pressure, causing short breathe, and desire for stool. Weakness of abdominal ring region. Forcing in lower abdomen towards genitals.

CARBO VEG: When Carbo veg is indicated, the digestion will be slow and imperfect, there will be weight in the stomach and bowels. There is burning in the stomach extending to the back and along the spine to the interscapular region. There is great distension of the stomach and bowels, which is temporarily relieved by belching. The flatulence of Carbo veg is found in the upper part of the abdomen. There is heaviness, fullness and sleepiness after eating. The symptoms are worse from fat, fish, oysters, ice-cream, vinegar or cabbage. Coffee disagrees, and milk increases the flatulence. There is violent burning in the stomach, chest and abdomen, with paroxysmal and crampy pains which force the patent to bend double. The patient wants to be fanned. It is useful remedy especially for the effects of overeating, high living or from eating tainted meats, where digestion being slow, the food putrefies before it digests. There is great craving for salt and other things, which makes him sick. There is upward pressure of gas on the diaphragm, causing distress of breathing.

CHINA OFFICINALIS: It is a remedy where problems are created due to loss of animal fluids. The distension of the stomach is painful and temporarily relieved by belching. There is sour or bitter eructation and the flatus is offensive, there is slow digestion and the patient faints easily. There is also a sensation as if food has lodged in the oesophagus behind the sternum. In china there is yellow diarrhoea, which is worse at night and after meals. In cases where the food does not digest, but lies a long time in the stomach, causing eructation's and finally is vomited undigested, China is the remedy.

LYCOPODIUM: It is suited for the chronic congestion and catarrhal conditions of the stomach in patients with liver and gouty troubles. There is great hunger but a few mouthfuls fill up to the throat. Distress immediately after eating, not a half-hour after. There is intolerance of pressure about the waist after meals. Patient is sleepy after eating. There is great accumulation of flatus especially in the lower part of the abdomen. Attacks of ravenous hunger are also found in Lycopodium. The patient is worse after late dinners, the distension lasting into the night, making him restless and waking at night. It is especially useful in atonic and acid forms of dyspepsia, for it has sour taste, sour belching and vomiting. The patient prefers hot drinks. There is desire for sweets.

PULSATILLA : Dryness of the mouth, putrid taste in the morning on awakening and a sensation as if food had lodged under the sternum are the important guiding symptoms of this remedy. The tongue is coated thick, rough, white fur, there is acidity and heartburn, food tastes bitter, sour and putrid, and there is water brash and eructation tasting of food and absence of thirst. There is craving for lemons and aversion to fats, which aggravate. There is often a constant taste of food on the mouth as if it had laid in the stomach a long time after eating it. A bad taste in the mouth. About one or two hours after eating there is feeling of fullness and weight in the stomach which is relieved for a short time by eating. After meals there is violent palpitation. The patient is active mentally, which keeps him awake late in the night.

□□□

CHAPTER 24

Headache

Headache is the most common of all nervous complaints. The causes are varied and so also its mode of onset, duration, intensity and other conditions associated with it.

Structures of the head, which are sensitive to pain, are:

i) All extra cranial coverings are pain sensitive, especially the scalp muscles and arteries.

ii) Of the intracranial structures, great venous sinuses and tributaries from the surface of the brain, parts of dura at the base, dural arteries and cerebral arteries at the base of the brain, the 5th, 9th and the 10th cranial nerves and upper three cervical nerves are pain sensitive.

iii) Pathways of pain from structure on or above the superior surface of the tentorium cerebelli are contained in the 5th cranial nerve. Pain is mostly in the fronto-temporo parietal region and within and behind the eyes. Paths for pain from those below the tentorium cerebelli are chiefly in the 9th and 10th cranial and upper 2 or 3 cervical nerves. The pain is felt in the auricular, post auricular and the occipital region.

Intracranial diseases cause headache mostly by involvement of more than one of the pain sensitive structures. Traction, displacement, distension and in certain cases inflammation of the cranial vascular structures or direct pressure by a cranial tumor on the pain producing nerves are chiefly responsible.

Thus, distension and dilatation of the intracranial arteries cause headache during fever, foreign protein allergy, sepsis, bactreamia, nitrite and carbon monoxide poisoning and asphyxia also causes headache following an epileptic attack, sudden high rise of blood pressure or headache of migraine or hypertensive crisis or of emotional state.

a) Primary intracranial lesions are neoplasm, meningitis and following lumbar puncture.

b) Painful conditions in the jaw or neck may be referred to the head.

c) Extra cranial arteries by stretch and dilatation or inflammation may cause pain.

d) Sustained contraction of the muscles of the scalp and neck is an important added factor in migraine.

e) Inflammations or other disturbances in the eye, ear, nose, teeth and scalp may cause headache.

NEURALGIA & HEADACHE: These two have certain points of resemblance but neuralgia has a special distribution, pain is intense and paroxysmal, has tender spots and may have an exciting peripheral cause.

Classification

1. *Local causes:* frontal sinusitis, sinus suppuration, the area is tender on pressure, nasal discharge is present, ski gram and transillumination are additional helps, head injury, osteitis, cervical fibrositis.
2. *Referred pain:* Nose, coryza, and deviated sputum. Eye error of refraction, more commonly myopic astigmatism (the pain is aggravated by eye strain and relieved by rest), iritis and glaucoma. Dental inflammation - otitis media. Gastric or utero-ovarian reflex.
3. *Nervous causes:* Neuralgias, especially trigeminal. The pain is wide spread or limited to the supraorbital region. Cerebral causes as meningitis, neoplasm, abscess, intercranial aneurysm, raised or lower intracranial pressure.
4. *Constitutional causes:* chronic nephritis, uraemia, too high or low blood pressure, polycythaemia, also severe anemia and congestive heart failure. Post epileptic condition, hysteria or psycogenic headache and migraine. Acute and chronic alcoholism, cyclic vomiting in children. Sea or aeroplane sickness, hypoxemia. Gastritis, chronic constipation, chronic hepatitis, diabetes mellitus, gout, lead poisoning. Acute fevers, especially malaria, enteric fever, small pox, scarlet fever, typhus, yellow fever and influenza.

Several of these cause pain in the vertex: these are hysteria, hypertension and heat stroke. Occipital headache is caused by meningitis, cerebral- spinal syphilis, cerebella tumour, chronic nephritis, myalgia and neuralgia.

Homoeopathic Medicines

BELLADONNA : It is the first remedy that comes into mind for headache. Throbbing is the great keynote of this remedy. But violent shooting pains in head, driving the patient crazy are but characteristic. The patient cannot lie down, must sit up, nor can he bear light or a draft of air, noise or jarring. The location of the pain is mostly in the frontal region or right side, flushed face, dilated pupils are also present. The headache of Belladonna is usually worse in the afternoon, the whites of the eyes are red, and the cornea is glassy, and moving eyes aggravate. The face is puffed and red. The headache is violent, pounding, throbbing, relieved by cold applications or having the head high. The face is flushed, the pulse full and bounding. Vertigo with falling to left side or backwards. Sensitive to least contact. Much throbbing and heat. Headache from suppressed catarrhal flow. : This is the remedy for the young, plethoric, usually healthy, patient.

NUX VOMICA : It is more often indicated in headache than any other remedy. Headache due to excessive use of alcohol, headache from digestive troubles, constipation, and especially from abuse of purgatives. It suits the gouty and haemorrhoidal patients. The pain is situated over the left eye or in the occiput. It begins in the morning with giddiness on first rising, and last all day until night and is accompanied with sour taste or nausea and violent retching. The dull, wooden, bursting feeling of the head following a debauch is the characteristic symptoms. The complexion looks muddy and the whites of the eyes are yellow and the urine is scanty and high coloured. Stooping and coughing aggravate the headache; it is worse in the morning; moving the eyes and motion in general makes the head feel worse. Headache is better by wrapping the head and by rest. It is a remedy to be given while the patient is still under the influence of liquor or any of the stages of alcoholism.

GELSEMIUM : It is the remedy, which has a headache commencing with blindness and it, is especially a remedy for headaches due to eyestrain. The pain in the Gelsemium begins in the occiput or nape of the neck, comes up over the head and settles in the eye. There is a feeling as if a band was about the head, the patient is dull and apathetic, and there is a great sensation in the eyes when moving them. Occipital headache, which are dull and dragging. Copious urination relieves the headache and headache is accompanied with visual troubles such as double vision, squinting and dim sight. Headache is relieved by sleep and dizziness may accompany the troubles. A characteristic of Gelsemium is a sensation of a band around the head just above the ears. It also suits the tobacco headache.

NATRUM MUR: The headache of Natrum Mur is as if there were little hammers beating in the skull, worse from moving the head or eyeballs. It comes on in the morning, is worse about 10 a.m. and is preceded by partial blindness. Earthy complexion of the face. Patient is irritable and gets into a passion about trifles. Wants to be alone to cry. Tears with laughter. Great weariness and weakness. Anaemic headache of schoolgirls. Chronic headache, semi lateral, congestive, from sunrise to sunset, with pale face, nausea and vomiting. Frontal sinus inflammation.

CIMICIFUGA: This is another remedy for the neuralgic form of headache. It corresponds to headache of students and those exhausted by fatigue. There is first a sensation as of top of the head would fly off. There are sharp, stitching and lancinating pains over the eyes, shooting to the top of the head. The brain seems to move in waves, and there may be the symptoms of a sharp pain extending from the occiput to the frontal region, as if a bolt were driven through the head. Headache due to some uterine irritation. When there is a feeling that the patient would go crazy it is especially indicated. Many of the pains begin in the occiput and shoot down the spine; there is a tendency to bend the head forward, which relieves somewhat.

CHAPTER 25

High Blood Cholesterol

Cholesterol is present in the diet of all people, and it can be absorbed slowly from the gastrointestinal tract into the intestinal lymph. It is highly fat soluble but only slightly soluble in water and is capable of forming esters with fatty acids.

Factors that affect plasma cholesterol concentration. The important factors that affect plasma cholesterol concentration are as follows:

1. An increase in the amount of cholesterol ingested each day increases the plasma concentration slightly.
2. A highly saturated fat diet increases blood cholesterol concentration 15 to 20 percent
3. Ingestion of fat containing highly unsaturated fatty acids usually depresses the blood cholesterol concentration in slight to moderate amount.
4. Lack of insulin or thyroid hormone increases the blood cholesterol concentration, whereas excess thyroid hormone decreases the concentration.

Normal blood cholesterol varies between 150 -200 mgm per 100 ml, which is equally distributed between plasma and corpuscles. But in the corpuscles it is present chiefly in the free form, while in the plasma the major part remains as esters. The rise of blood cholesterol is accompanied with the rise in bile cholesterol. There is also rise in blood cholesterol when cholesterol rich diet is not ingested which indicates that this is due to increased absorption of cholesterol derived from bile.

Arteriosclerosis or atherosclerosis has been observed in man fed with diet containing high cholesterol. In hypothyroidism blood cholesterol rises. In diabetes mellitus and atherosclerosis, blood cholesterol is often found to be high.

The factor most important in causing atherosclerosis is a high blood plasma concentration of cholesterol in the form of low-density lipoproteins. The plasma concentration of these high cholesterol low-density lipoproteins is directly increased by increased saturated fat in the daily diet. To a lesser extent, it is also increased by increased cholesterol in the diet. Therefore, both or either of these dietary factors can contribute to the development of atherosclerosis.

Familial hypercholesterolemia is a hereditary disease in which the person inherits defective genes for the formation of low-density lipoproteins receptors on the membrane surfaces of the body cells. In the absence of these receptors, the liver cannot reabsorb either the intermediate density lipoproteins or the low-density lipoproteins. Without this normal redelivery of cholesterol to the liver cells, the cholesterol machinery of the liver cells goes on a rampage producing new cholesterol, no longer responsive to the feedback inhibition of too much plasma cholesterol. As a result the number of very low density lipoproteins released by the liver into the plasma increases greatly, and the patient with full blown familial hypercholesterolemia will have a blood cholesterol concentration of 600 to 1000 mg/ dl, a level four to six times normal. Almost all these people die before the age of 20, some as early as 4 to 6, because of myocardial infarction or other sequel of atherosclerotic blockage of blood vessels through out the body.

A very good treatment is available in homoeopathy system of medicine for high blood cholesterol, which is given as under:

Homoeopathic Medicines

ACONITE: It has a marked influence on the heart. Numbness of the left arm; it also has tingling in the fingers, associated with heart disease. Aconite produces a cardiac congestion, with anxiety, oppression and palpitation, worse when walking, lancinating stitches occur and also attacks of intense pain. It is the remedy in uncomplicated hypertrophy of the heart. In pericarditis and endocarditis when the inflammation sets in with fever with the intense mental anxiety. There is great restlessness, tossing about, anxiety and fear of death. There is suddenness of onset of the symptoms and especially in young and plethoric persons who are full of life and vigour. Constant pressure in left chest; oppressed breathing on least motion.

CRATEGUS : This is a new remedy, and useful when the heart's action is feeble and irregular and the pulse small and intermittent; sensation as if heart would stop. It suits cases of failing compensation with dilatation of the heart and also fatty hearts. It acts well in functional diseases of heart, palpitation and tachycardia dependent upon anemia. In threatened heart failure during acute diseases it will work very well. Exhausting overwork. Nervous shock and neuroasthenia are usual symptoms. There is a painful sensation of pressure in the left side of the chest below the clavicle. It can be used as a tonic for weak heart.

DIGITALIS: The patient feels that the heart will stop beating if he should make any motion. This uneasy feeling about the chest rarely amounts to real pain. The digitalis patient has a doughy look to the skin; there is often a sick feeling at the stomach after eating. Disturbed sleep, apprehensive, deep, sighing, slow respiration, dry cough, suffocative spells. : It is known chiefly for its action on heart. The pulse is slow, but primarily strong, there is great weakness of the cardiac tissue and secondarily the pulse becomes weak. Extra exertion increased its rapidity but decreases its force, so that the quick pulse becomes irregular and intermittent. The heart feels as if the blood stood still. There is weakness and numbness of the left arm, and often blueness of the surface of the body, or cyanosis. It is also indicated in dropsical constitution dependent on heart trouble, swelling of feet and ankles, anasarca, cardiac dropsy associated with slow pulse, urine suppressed or scanty. Inflammation of the heart muscles coming slowly and in sudden cases of myocarditis or endocarditis.

KALMIA: Kalmia is an excellent remedy for cardiac troubles when they have been caused by the suppression of rheumatism by external applications. The pulse is slow. The sharp pains taking away the breath calls for this remedy. It is the remedy for cardiac hypertrophy, especially after rheumatism. Numbness of the left arm. There is much pain and anguish about the heart, some dsypnoea, palpitation and pressure from the epigastrium towards the heart. The heart is irregular and intermits every third or fourth beat. There are shooting pains through the chest to the scapula.

SPIGELIA: Heart symptoms accompany neuralgia. Irregular and tumultuous action of the heart. At times the heartbeat is audible. Rheumatic endocarditis will often be cured by this remedy. It has the most beneficial action in the angina pectoris. It corresponds well to chronic affections of the heart, particularly valvular disease and hypertrophy. There is palpitation worse from any movement of the arm or body. There is a purring sensation felt over the cardiac region when placing the hand thereon. The pulse is intermittent, not synchronous with the heartbeat, and the slightest motion of the arm or hands makes the patient worse. It is the remedy for the painful affections about the heart. There are sharp pains shooting from the heart to the back, and radiating from the heart down the arm, over the chest, and down the spine.

□□□

CHAPTER 26

How to Stop Smoking

Many thousands of people today are heavy smokers, not by choice, but because they have found no way of escape. They are caught in the grip of a habit developed during their teen-age years when so many young people think it is 'smart ' to smoke.

The strange thing is that most of these people never wanted to smoke in the first place. There was only doing what they thought everyone else was doing at the time. Yet there is another odd thing. Smoking in not a normal habit. A person has to learn to smoke.

Smoking is by and large, an acquired habit. People start smoking because they think it is fashionable to do so or because their friends and companions are able to persuade them to start smoking. Some smokers feel that they look more attractive to the opposite sex when they are smoking. Others hold that a social gathering becomes more intimate if people are smoking. In reality all this is a product of smokers imagination. Because he wants to justify his habit, he invents enough reasons for it.

According to the U.S. Health Authorities smoking is "the largest preventable cause of death in America." Millions of deaths are caused every year around the world by the smoking of cigarettes, pipes and cigars. Smoking causes coronary heart disease, lung cancer and skin cancer.

Why should we worry about smoking? For several reasons. Smoking is not merely an expensive luxury; it plays a definite part in lowering a person's resistance to disease. Heavy smokers die from 5 to 10 years earlier than non-smokers. In most cases the trouble is due to some condition of the heart or blood vessels. Another important factor is cancer of the lung.

Every cigarette a person smoke leaves him a little weaker and less able to carry on. Then why don't they stop? Because they are addicted to nicotine, a powerful drug that is present in the tobacco leaves. Some people seem to have little difficulty in giving up the habit, but most people have a real struggle. The majority continues to smoke because they get a temporary lift from the tobacco. However, this is always followed by a letdown, which then calls for another smoke.

Imagine the inside of a chimney or of an Indian tandoor. It is covered with black soot. Likewise our respiratory system including the most vital lungs are coated internally with unwelcome soot from cigarette smoke. The lung alveoli where the gaseous exchange takes place and the airways for the respiratory system are not designed for this sort of over-wrap. Thus smoking reduces the intake of clean air in to the respiratory system. The quantity of oxygen, which ought to go into he blood stream, is reduced and this produces an adverse effect on the brain as well as the heart.

Those who smoke pipes and cigars run the risk of developing lip and mouth cancer. The social impact of smoking is no less evil than its effect on the heart and the lungs. By way of personal hygiene, the smoker is at a disadvantage. His fingers turn yellow. His teeth and gums are stained. No mouthwash is enough to freshen his mouth.

How to Stop

How can a person actually stop smoking? Naturally the first thing to do is to stop. Whether a person decide to stop for just an hour at a time during the first day, or two hours the next and three hours the next day. Almost every smoker who genuinely wishes to stop will have a real struggle to face. What should one do? Here are a few steps one can take.

1. *Stay away* from other smokers as much as possible, particularly the next few weeks. This will reduce temptation and strengthen to resolve not to start again.
2. *Become a vigorous campaigner* against the use of tobacco in any form. This may bore some of your friends for a while, but in the end you may be able to help them too.
3. *Take two hot baths every day* and follow them with stimulating cold showers. This will help you physically and strengthen your will to succeed.
4. *Take plenty of exercise* including deep breathing and long walks in the open air several times each day. This will clean out the lungs and improve your sense of well being.

5. *Watch your diet.* Be sure to take large quantities of fresh fruits and vegetables. These are an excellent antidote against the poisons of tobacco. Infact, if you were to eat little except fruit and vegetables for the next few weeks you would soon lose your desire to smoke. If necessary take small meals more frequently to stabilize your blood sugar. This will also help to calm your nerves during this time of stress.
6. *Don't go hungry for long.* Eat regularly and do not attempt to lose weight while you are trying to break the tobacco habit. You may gain a few pounds, but don't worry about this just now. You can lose it later if need be.
7. *Avoid highly seasoned foods,* alcohol, tea and coffee. These have probably encouraged your craving for tobacco. They have spoiled your appetite for normal foods that build the body. Omit such things as pepper, mustard, spices, and all hot condiments from your diet. For the present you should even be careful about taking excessive amounts of salt. Drink at least ten glasses of water a day the first week. Taking a drink helps to reduce the craving for tobacco. If you will follow these instructions you will soon be surprised at the new flavors you are discovering in your foods.
8. *Get rid of all your cigarettes* and every vestige of tobacco you possess. It is not safe to keep any smoking materials handy just now. The temptation to start using the stuff may prove too great.
9. *Commit yourself to God* every day and every hour, asking Divine help whenever you feel the craving to smoke. Power from above is always available to those in need.
10. *Do not falter in your resolve* to conquer this habit, for it is well worth all the effort you will be forced to make.

Once you have solved this problem you will be surprised at how much better you feel. Your heart will beat quietly, your nerves will be calm and your muscles relaxed and your mind will be in control of itself. This will give you new moral and intellectual power, for you are no longer enslaved by a filthy habit. From now on you will enjoy better health and under the blessing of God, you will know true satisfaction and happiness.

Homoeopathic Medicines

NUX VOMICA: It corresponds to the tremor, to the nervous affections, to the headache, to the bad taste. It also corresponds to delirium tremens, where every little noise frightens and the victim finds no rest in any place, springs up at night and has frightful visions. The tremor is marked with ugliness and irritability and gastric disturbance. It is the right remedy for the acute results of a spree; the morning big head is often large enough for the Nux cap, and the "rich brown" taste corresponds beautifully. It is a remedy to be given while the patient is still under the influence of liquor or any of the stages of alcoholism.

CALADIUM SEGUINUM: It modifies craving for tobacco. Headaches and mental states of smokers. Very forgetful, does not know about the occurrences of things. Confused headache with pain shoulder, pressure in eyes and forehead; extremely sensitive to noise, throbbing in ear. This remedy has a marked action on the genital organs, and purities of this region. Coldness of single parts and inclination to lie down, with aggravation on lying on left side. Slightest noise startles from sleep. Dread from motion. Modifies craving for tobacco. Tobacco heart. Asthmatic complaints.

PHOSPHORUS: Partial loss of vision from abuse of tobacco. Phosphorus irritates, inflames and degenerates mucous membranes, irritates, and inflames serous membranes, inflames spinal cord and nerves, causing paralysis, destroys bone, especially the lower jaw and tibia; disorganizes the blood, causing fatty degeneration of blood vessels and every tissue and organs of the body and thus gives rise to haemorrhages.

Produces a picture of destructive metabolism. Causes yellow atrophy of the liver and sub-acute hepatitis. Tall, slender persons, narrow chested, with thin, transparent skin, weakened by loss of animal fluids, with great nervous debility, emaciation seems to be under the special influence of Phosphorus. Congestion of lungs sharp stitches in chest respiration quickened oppressed tuberculosis in tall, rapidly growing young people.

❑❑❑

CHAPTER 27

Influenza

It is a contagious, infectious disease. It is of short duration usually sporadic, characterized by malaise, headache, severe pain in the body and catarrh of the respiratory passage.

Metrological conditions are predisposing causes. The bacillus of Pfeiffer is generally acknowledged to be the exciting cause. The bacilli enter the system through respiratory organs.

The disease is highly infectious. Incubation period is 1 or 2 days and one attack does not give any immunity, rather increases the susceptibility.

There is much discrepancy and disagreement among over authorities on the question. In a case of simple uncomplicated flu, but find no characteristic anatomical lesions other than congestion and catarrhal secretions of the mucous membranes of the respiratory and alimentary systems. Death is usually caused by some complication and post-mortems show all the changes found in the complicating diseases.

Important symptoms are: chilliness; aching of muscles, eyeballs; bones; temperature high and low; delirium; prostration, usually marked and rapid; hemorrahages from nose, lungs, uterus; face pale or flushed and besotted; discharges from the mucous membranes, watery, bloody, mucous, purulent or mixed, bland or acrid, scanty or profuse; thick or thin, and of all colours; myalgias and neuralgias. We meet all the modalities of position, time of day and temperature.

When we have pneumonia or bronchitis as complications. Cough of every variety from an extremely dry and croupy to a lose catarrhal; expectoration of mucus, blood, mucus, pus and occasionally pure blood; rales of every variety. Profuse gelatinous exudates, which filled the lungs and choked the patient to death. Of the muscles, those of the heart seemed to suffer most. The pulse varied greatly and in many cases the hearts action failed completely, after being hard, soft, regular or irregular, slow or rapid, etc. Although, these are the few leading symptoms of the disease.

Some of the important homoeopathic medicines are given below: -

Homoeopathic Medicines

GELSEMIUM: When sneezing, frequent and violent; chilliness up and down the back; face flushed dark red, a free watery discharge from the nostrils, usually non-irritating; a dull, heavy aching of the muscles. No thirst; great prostration and marked trembling; pulse full but soft; listless, apathetic. Gelsemium is the best homoeopathic medicine. The patient is dull and weak, chills run up and down the back, with a watery, excoriating, or bland discharge from the nose and sneezing. General weakness. Dizziness, drowsiness, dullness and trembling. Slow pulse tired feeling, mental apathy. Muscular weakness. Complete relaxation and prostration. Lack of muscular coordination. Fullness of the head, hot fever and chilliness as if a cold were coming on. The patient is dull and weak, chills run up and down the back, with a watery, excoriating, or bland discharge from the nose and sneezing. There is also a marked inclination in the patient to hug the fire. Cold brought on by warm relaxing weather indicate Gelsemium, hence it seems to be, most useful in spring and summer weather. There is a predisposition to take cold on any change of weather. It has been extremely useful in influenza with fever

ARSENICUM: The patient is extremely restless; the chills alternate with the fever; there is violent thirst, but both food and drinks are soon vomited, i.e., the stomach is very irritable, there is violent sneezing and discharge from the nose which is very acrid and excoriating; the stools are diarrheic; the urine scanty, often albuminous; the pains are burning in character but amel. by heat; the prostration is so great the patient can hardly move, he cannot remain quiet because he is restless; there is fear of death or if he recovers, he will never be able to do anything. There is dull, frontal headache and sneezing, photophobia, the sneezing does not relieve in the slightest and the irritation continues as before and is worse on going into the open air. Burning and bleeding. Acne of nose. The Arsenic patient is always fearful of the outcome of his condition. Great thirst drinks much but little at a time. Debility, exhaustion and restlessness with nightly aggravation are the leading indications for this remedy.

EUPATORIUM PERF : Eupatorium perf. cured old & weak people when there were chill followed by vomiting of bile; pain and soreness of eye balls, water tastes oily; great soreness and severe aching of bones and muscles; pain in the occiput after lying on it, with the sense of weight; coryza with sneezing; so that patient must support it with a hand amel. by binding chest tight, vomiting and purging of large amount of bilious, green and watery substance. Hoarseness and cough, with soreness in chest; must support it. Influenza with great soreness of muscles and bones. Chronic loose cough, chest sore, worse at night. Cough relieved by getting on hands and knees.

SABADILLA : Sneezing is the great keynote of this remedy. Sneezing and lacrymation on going into open air. The throat is swollen and the pain is worse on empty swallowing; the sneezing is excessive, shaking the whole body. Shuddering, with gooseflesh creeping upwards, are also prominent symptoms. Frontal headache, dryness of mouth, without thirst and cough, worse on lying down, are additional symptoms. It suits well to many cases of the catarrhal form of grippe. Coryza, with severe frontal pains and redness of eyes and lacrymation. Copious, watery nasal discharge. Sore throat; begins on left side. Dry fauces and throat. Sensation of a lump in throat with constant desire to swallow. Chronic sore throat; worse from cold air.

ALLIUM CEPA: The nasal discharge is thin and flows constantly, excoriates the upper lip, and there is prolonged sneezing. The discharge ceases when the patient goes into the open air, but returns when entering a warm room again. It is a drug which should be given early, and if there be a splitting laryngeal cough, causing the patient to wince and crouch it is indicated. Feeling of a lump at the root of nose. Fluent coryza with headache, cough and hoarseness. : It is one of the best remedies for cold in the head. The discharge is profuse, thin and acrid, with great smarting in the nose and eyes. There is profuse lacrymation, which is bland. The edges of the eyelids burn and the eyes are red and sensitive to light.

NUX VOMICA : The nose is dry, there is very little discharge, the eyes are watery and there is scraping in the throat, and dullness and oppression about the front sinuses; it should be given as soon as dryness and tickling in the nose begins; the nasal passages are alternately free and obstructed. These symptoms are worse in a warm room and better in the open air. It is of little use when the cold is fully developed. Nose is stuffed up at night. Odors tend to produce fainting. Coryza fluent in daytime; stuffed up at night and outdoors; or alternates between nostrils. Bleeding in morning. Acrid discharge, but with stuffed up feeling. Tickling after waking in the morning. Sensation of roughness, tightness and tension. Nux vomica has colds caused by cold weather, with a dry, stuffed up nose and rough, scrappy throat. The first stage of ordinary cold in the head may be cured by Nux Vomica, when it is brought on by damp, cold weather, or from sitting on damp, cold steps, associated with sneezing and stuffed up feeling in the nose.

❑❑❑

CHAPTER 28

Insomnia

Inability to go to sleep or to get sleep for a period insufficient for the needs of an individual is known as insomnia. Chronic inability to sleep.

None of us can do without sleep. An infant sleeps 14 to 18 hours a day. This period is slowly reduced. An adult may be happy with 7 to 8 hours of sleep every night. There are people who require 5 hours or even 4 hours of sleep in 24 hours.

Sleep has a definite purpose and that is why all mammals sleep. Lack of sleep apparently does not cause any physical harm. But anyone who gets less than his normal sleep experiences a decrease of efficiency and concentration.

In old age, sleep normally becomes fitful. It is good to regulate sleeping hours. One should go to bed at a fixed time. The human body maintains a 24-hour cycle. During this cycle, the body temperature rises and falls at fixed times. In the middle of the night, the body temperature comes down. In the afternoon, it reaches its maximum. It is comfortable to be sleeping when the body temperature is at its lowest. If someone were compelled to be awake by the circumstances at his time, he would not feel physically and mentally at his best.

The most common cause of insomnia is worry; the other is depression. Environmental disturbances also cause lack of sleep.

Loss of sleep often results in fatigue and quickly impairs a person's normal judgment. The higher centers of the brain are the first to show the effects of overwork and anxiety. Such a person may become depressed, losing all interest in life and burdened with a sense of impending death. Unreasonable fears now arise to the surface of his mind, causing all kinds of anxiety and distress, as well sensation of acute pain.

Sleeping pills should be avoided. Sleeping pills taken over a long period disturb the second phase of the normal sleep, the rapid eye movement phase and thus cause harm to the person consuming them. Moreover, the effect of the drugs may last beyond the normal time for waking up and thus cause a reduction in efficiency and concentration. Sleeping pills mixed with alcohol can even be fatal. Patient should practice some technique to relax. Yoga can help or listening to music.

Shakespeare in Macbeth said, "Sleep that knits up the ravell'd sleeve of care, the death of each day's life, sore labor's bath, Balm of hurt minds, great nature's second course, Chief nourisher in life's feast."

Homoeopathy offers harmless medicines for lack of sleep or insomnia. It may be good, however, not to overload the stomach with food before going to sleep. A heavy meal disturbs sleep. A bath before going to bed is of positive help and so is exercise in the afternoon. In order to get good sleep taking a cup of hot milk before going to bed is a useful habit.

Late nights affect health most adversely because, after 10:30 p.m., the body requires rest and sleep while a late dinner, social function or a musical evening running into morning hours disturb the sleep patterns which is most suitable to the human body.

Stimulants brews like coffee or tea should be avoided in the late evening. Coffee after dinner has an adverse effect on sleep. Smoking of cigarettes also stimulates and thus keeps sleep await.

The sleeping environment should be as comfortable as possible, neither too hot nor too cold. Beds, which are too soft, are not conducive to sound sleep. The bed should be firm, hard and of a proper size.

A few useful homoeopathic medicines are given below:

Homoeopathic Medicines

NUX VOMICA: The great characteristic of this remedy is that the patient is very sleepy in the evening, cannot keep awake; the sleep is not sound or restful and the patient is awakened at night by anxiety and frightful dreams. He awakens at about four or five o'clock in the morning feeling little refreshed, but soon resleeps and awakens at the usual time feeling worse than ever. It is especially the remedy for those who drink too much, those who abuse coffee and tea, those who are subject to abdominal disorders and a sluggish portal circulation. Sleeplessness from mental overworks, from too close study, especially at night. The morning sleep aggravates all the complaints. Drowsy after meals and in early evening. Dreams full of bustle and hurry. Better after a short sleep unless aroused.

COFFEA: In cases where there is excessive agitation of body and mind, and where ideas force themselves on the mind. The patient is wide-awake, without the slightest inclination to sleep, and all the senses are extremely acute. It is the remedy when excitement or good news, joys or night watching causes the insomnia. It is well suited to sleeplessness in teething children. Sleeplessness from the bad effects of too good news. Sleeps till 3 a.m. after which only dozing. Wakes with a start sleep disturbed by dreams. Sleepless, on account of mental activity; flow of ideas, with nervous excitability. Sleep disturbed by itching of anus.

HYOSCYAMUS: Sleeplessness from mental excitement; the brain is full of bewildering ideas and images. After long illnesses and the brain cells are ill nourished this remedy is useful. It is especially indicated in sleeplessness in children, who twitch, cry out frightened and tremble. Sleeplessness from overwork and without apparent cause.

CANNABIS INDICA: It is indicated in the obstinate and intractable forms of insomnia. Sleep is irregular. It produces a tranquil slumber, relieves the nervousness and neuralgic pains. Very sleepy but unable to do so. Dreams of dead bodies.

BELLADONNA: The sleepless conditions in Belladonna are due to congestion; sleep is extremely restless, as a rule talking, starting, muscular jerking and spasmodic motions interrupt it; frightful images appear on closing the eyes and the patient is therefore dreads sleep. Children awake from sleep frightened. Sometimes there is a violent throbbing in the brain, which prevents sleep. The dreams found under this remedy are frightful and they constantly awaken the patient. It is probably the best remedy for insomnia due to cerebral hyperaemia. It is also a useful remedy in restless sleep during dentition; sleeps with eyes partially open; sudden starting, twitching, hot head and pupils dilated. Sleeps with hands under head.

GELSEMIUM: For insomnia of brainworkers it is the remedy. It is indicated in businessmen who pass restless nights, awakens early in the morning and worry over their business affairs. It is also the most useful remedy in a state of alternate excitement and depression. Gelsemium also has sleeplessness from emotional disturbances, and after evening company. Sleeplessness from over exertion. Delirious on falling sleep. Sleepless from nervous irritation.

CHAPTER 29

Intestinal Worms

Worms and other intestinal parasites are found in every part of the world. They are more common in tropical and sub tropical areas and are more common during the rainy season. Most of these worms and parasites enter in the human body either through the mouth or through the skin of the feet.

Round worms, are the giant worms present in the intestines that cause the disease kwon as ascariasis. It is found in almost all the countries. These worms are off-white in colour, are long and thick and are most frequently seen in children. Eggs produced by them are passed in stools. When children play in the soil contaminated with the eggs, particularly children living under unhygienic conditions easily transfer them to the mouth via dirty fingers.

Roundworm eggs may remain alive in the soil for many months. There is always greater danger of contamination where human wastes are used in fertilizing vegetables. Great care must be taken to be sure all foods are thoroughly cleansed and sterilized by cooking before being used.

When the round worm eggs reach the duodenum or small bowel they quickly hatch. The young worms borrow into the intestinal wall and then migrate to the liver and from there to the heart and lungs, producing bronchitis. Later they reach the small intestines again where they develop into mature worms causing nausea and vomiting, loss of weight, fever, nervousness, and irritability. Many patients complain of colicky pains and diarhoea. A mass of writhing worms in the intestines may produce complete obstruction of the bowel.

The adult worms may migrate through the intestinal walls and cause severe peritonitis. They may find their way into other areas, causing appendicitis, gall-bladder trouble, and liver disease. When the worms die, they cause toxic reactions, such as swelling of the face, loss of appetite and severe nervous symptoms.

HOOKWORM: It is a serious disease caused by small worms, which attach themselves to the walls of the intestines. Within the bowel they cause serious bleeding, and poison the patient as well. Hookworm infections are found mainly in warm, moist areas of the tropics, but are also found in some temperate zones.

It is most frequent in rural areas where the soil is loose and sandy where there are improper sanitary facilities. The tiny larval forms passed into the soil via stools enter the body through bare foot causing local itching and inflammation. Then they enter the smaller blood vessels and are carried to the lungs where they make their way to one of the bronchial tubes and then down into the small intestine and finally develop into adult worms. As the worms pass through the lungs they cause severe bronchitis.

Hookworms may live in the body for several years. They feed mainly on the blood. They produce a toxin, which increased the bleeding produced by the bite of the worm.

Patients with hookworm disease appear pale and are weak. They complain of dizziness, ringing in the ears, headache and are easily fatigued. The hair is dry, and the facial expressions dull and apathetic. In severe cases the heart is enlarged, and there may be swelling in all the tissues of the body. Shortness of breath occurs on slightest exertion. Nausea and vomiting are frequent. Children may develop mental retardation and growth is also impaired. Women and men may develop impotency.

PINWORMS: These are small white worms about a quarter of an inch in length. It is also limited to rural areas like other intestinal infections. Children are the most affected but adults may also suffer from this disease.

The adult worms live in the upper part of the colon, feeding on the intestinal contents. Mature female worms store eggs in there body and then migrate out through the colon and rectum to the skin where they lay eggs. These eggs bring on intense itching, causing the patient to scratch in the area around the rectum so that the fingers under the nails pick many of the eggs up. From there they are transferred to the mouth and are swallowed. They hatch in the stomach and then migrate down to the lower bowel and in this way the cycle continues.

Some people have slight infections of pinworms without any noticeable symptoms. But others complain of severe itching around the anal areas, a poor appetite, and loss of weight, bed-wetting, sleeplessness, and irritability, grinding of teeth, nausea, and vomiting and even appendicitis in some cases. Pinworms sometimes migrate into the vagina and cause intense itching and inflammation of the female genital tract.

TAPEWORM INFECTIONS: These vary in size. Some tapeworms are only a few inches long; others measure from ten to thirty feet or more in length. Cattle may develop the disease by grazing on grass contaminated with human wastes and thus pick up the eggs of these parasites. Human contract the disease by eating incompletely cooked meat from such animals.

The clinical picture varies depending on how many worms are present in the bowel. Tapeworms are present for years without producing any symptoms. Some patients complain of hunger pain, which is sharp and stabbing but immediately relieved by eating. There may be some anaemia, which is cured when worms are removed.

Homoeopathic Medicines

CINA: It produces an exact picture of a wormy child. The patient is cross, irritable, has a sickly pale face with rings about the eyes, grinds the teeth at night and has a tendency to convulsions; there is canine hunger or variable appetite; the child picks at its nose and cries out in its sleep; there is jerking of the hands and feet and a milky urine. It does not correspond well to pinworms and a noticeable symptom is a bluish color about the mouth. The cina patient is hungry, cross, ugly and wants to be rocked. Skin sensitive to touch. Child very cross does not want to be touched, or carried. Desires many things but refuses when given. Itching of the anus. Twisting pain about the navel. Gets hungry soon after a meal. Hungry, digging, gnawing sensation. Vomiting and diarrhoea immediately after eating or drinking. Vomiting with a clean tongue. Craving for sweets.

STANNUM: It has many worm symptoms, pale and sunken face and eyes surrounded by blue rings. Sluggish disposition; general weakness. Patient prefers to lie on stomach. Hunger, smell of cooking causes vomiting. Bitter taste. Pain better by pressure but sore to touch. Sensation of emptiness in the stomach. Cramp like around the navel with a feeling of emptiness. Colic relieved by hard pressure.

SPIGELIA : Jerking with paleness of face, blue rings around the eyes, faint, nauseated feeling with colic about the navel caused by the presence of worms. Child refers to the navel as most painful part. Itching and crawling in the rectum. Frequent ineffectual urging for stool.

CALCAREA CARB : Stool large and hard whitish, watery, sour. Diarrhoea of undigested food, fetid with ravenous appetite. Constipation; stool at first hard, then pasty, then liquid. It is indicated for the children who grow fat, are large belied, with large head, pale skin, chalky look. Children crave eggs and eat dirt and other indigestible things. Its chief action is on the vegetative sphere. Increased local and general perspiration. Calcarea patient is fat, fair, flabby and perspiring. Swollen abdomen. Cannot tolerate tight clothing around the waist. Patient is worse from exertion, mental or physical. Anxiety with palpitation. Aversion to work or exertion. Loss of appetite when overworked. Cramps in stomach; worse pressure, cold water. Ravenous hunger. Swelling over pit of stomach, like a saucer turned bottom up. Pain in epigastric region. Thirst; longing for cold drinks.

CHAPTER 30

Jaundice

Jaundice is a disease marked by a yellow discoloration in the skin, or in the whites of the eyes. This is due to excessive amounts of bile in the blood stream. Jaundice may arise from a number of different causes. Some types of jaundice arise from conditions outside the liver. Also in some cases the patient may have jaundice in a sub clinical form. That is, the bile pigment may be elevated but not sufficiently to actually discolour the skin.

Normally there is a certain rate at which the red blood cell are broken down and destroyed in the body. The average life of a red cell is about four months. But certain disease conditions may cause an excessive breakdown of red cells and this increases the bile pigment in the blood. Such a rapid breakdown of cells may be seen in haemolytic anaemia, sickle cell anaemia, pernicious anaemia, jaundice of the newborn child, as well as in malaria, pneumonia, yellow fever and certain bacterial infections of the blood.

Obstructive jaundice means that the bile is backing up into the blood stream because of some obstruction involving the larger bile ducts. The normal liver produces one pint of bile every twenty-four hours. This is transported to the gall bladder where it is concentrated and becomes green, or else passes directly to the small intestine where it acts as a lubricant. Bile is also necessary for the absorption of fats and for its laxative effect in the large intestine.

Bile gives colour to the faeces. When it is absent, the stools become very light, almost white in colour. Anything that obstructs the flow of bile to the intestine will not only to produce light coloured stools but may also result in jaundice. The obstruction may be due to a stone or stricture in the bile ducts, or perhaps to hepatitis or cirrhosis of the liver, or even cancer in the head of the pancreas.

Stones in the common duct are a frequent cause of jaundice. The patient notes a sharp, sudden pain in the upper part of the abdomen near the midline. Fever soon develops, and after a few hours or days jaundice will usually appear. It is first seen in the whites of the eyes, later spreading to all the skin and mucous membranes of the body.

Jaundice is particularly common in the middle-aged ladies who have had several children. Jaundice due to cancer comes on more slowly, and there is little or no pain at the beginning. In either case the jaundice will continue until the obstruction is removed, may last for weeks or months, depending on the patient's general condition. In acute hepatitis, on the other hand, jaundice may appear quickly but usually subsides within a week or ten days.

The size of the liver is reduced from one to two-thirds the normal weight. This atrophy is in some cases preceded by hypertrophy. The capsule is shrunken and the colour is of a grayish- yellow hue. When cut we may have a red colour in the first stage but it becomes yellow in the later stages. The microscope reveals the destruction of the hepatic cells, generally beginning in the terminal veins. Fat globules with free pigment are found in the cell walls displacing the nuclei.

The first symptoms are those of catarrhal jaundice, the stomach symptoms being the most prominent. In the course of a few days the skin becomes intensely icterus. The subjective symptoms are general malaise, dull headache, anorexia and nausea. The objective symptoms are the profound icterus, the uncontrollable vomiting, the tongue dry and brown, the fever, the violent delirium, convulsions, sordes on the teeth and other typhoid manifestations.

Diagnosis is difficult during the first stage, but comparatively easy in the second. The rapidly increasing jaundice, the vomiting, the hemorrhages, the marked delirium and the large amount of bile in the urine with leucin and tyrosine, the tenderness as size of the liver decreases, gives us a very good picture which is rarely duplicated in any other disease.

Catarrhal jaundice and hypertrophic cirrhosis may be mistaken for it during the first stage, but the tenderness and size of the liver will differentiate from the first, and the fever and urinary symptoms from the latter.

Homoeopathic Medicines

BRYONIA: Stitching pain in the right hypochondriac region, Bryonia is the first to medicine to be thought of, Under Bryonia the liver is swollen, congested and inflamed; the pains in the hypochondriac region are worse from any motion, and better from lying on the right side, which lessens the motion of the parts when breathing. It is one of the chief remedies for jaundice brought on by a fit of anger. Patient is chilly. There is bitter taste in the mouth and the stools are hard and dry or if loose are profuse and associated with a colic. Bryonia is preeminently a gastro-hepatic remedy and has pain in the right shoulder, giddiness, skin and eyes slightly yellow. Liver region swollen, sore, tensive. Burning pain, stitches worse from pressure, coughing and breathing. Tenderness of abdominal walls. Thirst for large quantities of water. Pressure in stomach after eating as of a stone.

MERCURIUS: This remedy has much sensitiveness and dull pain in the region of the liver; the patient cannot lie on the right side. The liver is enlarged. The skin and conjunctiva are jaundiced. The stools are either clay coloured from absence of bile, or yellowish green bilious stools passed with a great deal of tenesmus. There is yellowish white-coated tongue, which imprint of the teeth and there is a foetid breath, loss of appetite and depression of spirits. Mercurius is the remedy for jaundice arising from abuse of quinine when fever is present. It is a splendid remedy for torpid liver. It suits well simple jaundice in children. General tendency to free perspiration but the patient is not relieved thereby.

PODOPHYLLUM : The principle use of Podophyllum is in the liver affections. Primarily it induces a large flow of bile, and secondarily, great torpidity followed by jaundice. It is indicated in torpid and chronically congested liver when diarrhoea is present. The liver is swollen and sensitive, the face and eyes are yellow and there is a bad taste in the mouth. The tongue is coated white or yellow and the bile may form gallstones. There is loose watery diarrhoea, or if constipation were present the stools are clay-coloured. Another symptom of Podophyllum is that the patient constantly rubs the region of the liver with the hand. There is constipation clay coloured stool, jaundice and languor. Thirst for large quantities of cold water. Diarrhoea of long standing; early in morning; during teething with hot glowing cheeks while being bathed or washed in hot whether after acid fruits.

CHELIDONIUM : The liver symptoms of Chelidonium are very prominent. There is soreness and stitching pains in the region of the liver, but the keynote for this drug in hepatic disease is a pain under the angle of the right shoulder blade, which may extend on the chest, stomach, or hypochondria; there is swelling of the liver, chilliness, fever, jaundice, yellow coated tongue, bitter taste and a craving for acids and sour things, such as pickles and vinegar. The stools are profuse, bright yellow and diarrhoeic; they may be clayey in colour. It is a remedy to be used in simple biliousness and jaundice, and in hepatic congestion or inflammation. It causes the liver to secrete thinner and more profuse bile than any other remedy. It is useful remedy to promote the expulsion of the gallstones, and to prevent their formation. In simple catarrhal jaundice it is often all sufficient. It mainly affects the left lobe of the liver.

NUX-VOMICA : In liver affections occurring in those who have indulged in excess of alcoholic liquors, highly seasoned food, quinine, or in those who have abused themselves with purgatives, Nux is the first remedy to be thought of. The liver is swollen hard and sensitive to the touch and pressure of clothing. The first remedy in the cirrhosis of liver. Colic may be present. Jaundice induced by the anger, from abuse of quinine. Liver engorged with stitches and soreness. Colic with upward pressure, causing short breathe and desire for stool. Weakness of abdominal ring region. Alternate constipation and diarrhoea after abuse of purgatives. Diarrhoea with jaundice.

LYCOPODIUM : It acts powerfully on the liver. The region of the liver is sensitive to touch and there is a feeling of tension in it, a feeling as if a cord were tied about the waist. Cirrhosis. Fullness in the stomach after eating a small quantity. There is apt to be weight and aching in the liver, he can lie on that side, but no turning to the left side, the liver seems to pull and draw. Lycopodium is more useful than any other remedy in old hepatic congestions. Pain in right side and back from congestion will often lead to this remedy.

□□□

CHAPTER 31

Kidney Stones

The common stones found in the kidneys are of calcium oxalate, uric acid, urates, triple phosphates or a combination of these.

The patients are often males between 30 to 50 years.

a) Hot dry climate, retardation of free urinary flow and infection, disordered metabolism and hyperparathyroidism are the predisposing factors. The stone is formed in concentrated urine having perceptible crystalloids and in addition a colloid binding substance as fibrin, mucus, pus and cellular debris.

b) Reaction of the urine is important for the crystallization. A hyperacid urine having Ph of 5 is favorable for precipitation of uric acid and alkaline urine of pH 8, for phosphates and carbonates

c) An infection supplies the colloid required.

The size and the appearance of the stones vary: may be much small sand like particles or big oval or branching calculi nearly filling the renal pelvis. The oxalate stone is more common and is rough, hard and spiny may have a coating of altered blood. The uric acid stone is brown, hard and on section has a laminated appearance. The phosphate stone is white, soft and chalky and may sometimes be deposited on the urate or oxalate stone.

The stones may remain in the renal pelvis and increase in size. These exert pressure on the kidney, causing atrophy, also erosion and perinephritic abscess. If the stone reaches the bladder, irritation and infection may follow, the urine may become alkaline and the stone becomes bigger and encrusted with phosphates.

The symptoms depend upon the shape, size and position of the stones. A smooth small one may travel the whole passage without symptoms. A stone fixed in one of the calyces without infection may remain latent for years. There may be either no symptoms or only a dull ache in the loin, aggravated by the movements especially by jolting, of the same and rarely of the opposite side; slight albuminuria, haematuria and sometimes polyuria are present in some cases. But when a small stone passes down to enter the ureter and is big enough to block it, more obvious indication is paroxysmal attacks of renal colic.

Colic is characterized by sudden severe pain often following muscular exercise especially riding, starts from the lumbar region and following the distribution of the genitocrural nerve, runs downwards along the Pouparts ligament into the thigh and the scrotum or labium majus in female. The patient is in intense agony during paroxysm, tosses in bed, bathed in cold sweat and he vomits frequently. This continues for several minutes or hours and often disappears as suddenly: oxalates tones being harder and rougher, cause most severe pain. The parts involved in pain continue to be hyperalgesic for sometime afterwards.

There is frequent desire for urination but the urine is scanty, high coloured and even contains blood. Occasionally crystals of stone are passed. If there is infection, fever and leucocytosis are also present. In case of complete block of the ureter, if the other kidney is grossly diseased or its function reflexly inhibited, there may be anuria.

Later, the calculus reaching the bladder may cause vesicle irritability and pain at the root of the penis and perineum after micturition.

In a favorable case, the stone may be passed out without further relapse of the colic but more often multiple stones are present and attacks are repeated for several years.

Complications are pyelitis, pyelonephritis, cystitis, and extravasations of urine through ulcerated ureter, hydronephrosis, anuria, progressive renal fibrosis, uraemia and sometimes-malignant disease.

The ureter of the pelvis may be periodically or partially blocked causing hydronephorosis occasionally pyonephrosis. Progressive renal insufficiently may develop or there may be sudden block of the ureters causing complete anuria and death from uraemia.

Diagnosis is made by (i) the history of renal colic (ii) Urinary deposits show blood, pus and crystals of the stone, (iii) X-ray picture of both the kidneys and also of the bladder: oxalates give the best shadow and cystine very little. Uric acid stone is somewhat transparent but gives shadow if encrusted with lime salts. Renal colic without a calculus shadow may be due to a blood clot or cellular debris. (iv) Pyelography is also necessary (this differentiates shadow of the stone from the same of a calcified lymphatic gland)

Renal colic is to be differentiated from (a) other colic as biliary, appendicular, intestinal or pancreatic, (b) other renal diseases as torsion, tuberculosis, infraction, new growth or(c) genitocrural neuralgia.

Prognosis is not immediately bad provided urinary sepsis is attended to and urinary flow is copious and gross structural changes in the kidneys have not taken place.

Homoeopathic Medicines

CANTHARIS: It is the first remedy required for a urinary difficulty. There is persistent and violent urging to urinate, with great tenesmus; the urine is passed through the urethera, burning is very intense. There is aching in the small of back. It is often indicated in acute cystitis; gravel and uretheritis, important symptoms being the burning and the tenesmus of the bladder; haemuturia also calls for this remedy. There is constant urging to urinate, even small amount of urine in the bladder bringing the urging, which is accompanied by the terrible distress at the neck of the bladder. In the region of the kidneys there is cutting pain, which extends to the abdomen, the bladder and urethra. The pain is aggravated immediately following urination. The urine itself under Cantharis is of a deep red color, deposits sediment of mucus and often contains fibrinous cast.

APIS MELLIFICA : The most important symptoms for Apis in urinary infections are scanty or suppressed urine, drowsiness, and oedema in various parts, thirstlessness and suffocation on lying down. The urine is dark, highly albuminous, and contains casts. In difficult micturition of Apis is a useful remedy. It has a frequent desire, with the passage of few drops at a time. There is great irritation at the neck of the bladder and incontinence of urine. Burning and soreness when urinating. Urine is suppressed loaded with casts; frequent and involuntary, stinging pain and strangury. Last drops burn and smart. Swelling or puffing up of various parts, oedema, red rosy hue, stinging pains, soreness, intolerance of heat, and slightest touch, and afternoon aggravation are some of the important guiding symptoms.

BERBERIS VULGARIS : It is one of the principle remedies for genitourinary organs. It has a severe tearing pain in the kidneys, not only in the back but also deep in the kidneys themselves, these pains extend down the back and down the ureters into the bladder, cutting pains in the bladder extending into the urethra. These pains in the back and along the urethra are very severe; they are worse stooping, lying or sitting and relieved by standing. In the bladder they cause a desire to urinate, and the patient is constantly urinating, for the bladder seems imperfectly emptied. There is pain in the bladder. The urine is reddish, deposits consisting of mucus, epithelium and lithates. There is pain in the hips while urinating.

NUX VOMICA : It powerfully affects the urinary organs. It affects the lower part of the spine. There is incontinence of urine and irritability at the neck of the bladder. There is frequent ineffectual urging to urinate and burning and tearing pains accompany these, the urine passes in drops. There is paralysis of the bladder. There is dribbling or retention of urine. Haematuria from abuse of drugs. Cystitis with this painful urging and scanty urine indicates the remedy. The straining is violent at times, and the urine is dark with red brick dust sediment, or bloody or mixed with tenacious mucus.

□□□

CHAPTER 32

Low Back Pain

Most backaches seem to begin while bending forward to pick up some object from the floor. The pain usually comes on suddenly without warning, and it may be very difficult to straighten up to a standing position again. In most cases it is felt either in the middle of the back or lower down on one side. If a spinal disc is involved, the pain may radiate down the thigh and leg along the sciatic nerve on that side. The most common cause of backache probably arises from failure to get enough exercise to keep the muscles of the back strong and healthy. Flabby muscles then produce a wobbly spine, followed by pain, spasm and misery especially if a disc is ruptured.

Weakened muscles and damaged discs are not the only causes of low back pain. There are many more, such as menstruation, pregnancy, female disorders, kidney and bladder conditions, as well as rectal and prostatic diseases. Usually these bring little or no pain on moving the back. In this they differ from a weakened back in which movement is always painful.

Another condition known as osteoporosis, or thinning of the bones, is often seen in elderly people. This may cause collapse and wedging of one or more of vertebrae, owing to the weakening of the bones, which often occurs in the later years of life. Such conditions need careful medical management to prevent further deformity and pain. Many patients suffering from the disease have benefited by controlled use of male and female hormone tablets or injections. They should be given a good diet, including sufficient protein and calcium to restore the tissues of the bones.

Arthritis of the spine is another common cause of low back pain. Fractures of the spine often result in severe back pain. A qualified surgeon who can prescribe any appliances or supports that may be needed should treat such conditions.

Avoid Back Trouble

Most backaches could be avoided following a few simple rules:

1. *Lift with legs,* not the back. Bend your knees when you wish to pick up something heavy. Keep the back straight.
2. *Avoid overexertion.* A person who is not accustomed to heavy lifting should not try to carry too much at a time.
3. *Exercise regularly.* Don't overdo a good thing like exercise. Taking a moderate amount regularly will do more good than strenuous exercise on rare occasions.
4. *Change your position frequently.* Avoid cramped sitting positions that bring on fatigue. Move around. Keep flexible.
5. If you do have back trouble, *do not worry.* With proper treatment your back will soon be better.

Sprained Back

A sprained is the result of a bending or overextension of a joint beyond its normal range. Any unexpected twisting of the body, such as in car accident, may cause a badly sprained back. But merely bending over to pick up one's shoes may also produce a sudden "catch" of pain in the middle of the back, making it difficult to straighten up again. During the next or two the pain becomes worse and the nearby muscles go into spasm. All movements must then be restricted to prevent further pain.

Regular exercise is important. As soon as the pain begin to subside, the patient should lie on the floor with his hands behind the neck and raise the legs high in the air. First one at time, then together. Repeat this a dozen times each morning and night. Careful bending from side to side and also rotating the upper part of the body while holding the lower part steady will help to strengthen the back and keep the muscles strong and vigorous. At the same time it will restore tone to all tendons, ligaments and joints.

Homoeopathic Medicines

RHUS TOX : A violent pain in the back, as if broken, is the greatest characteristic of Rhus tox. It is more characteristic that the pain is relieved from motion. It is especially suitable to affections of the deeper muscles of the back. There are great pains, dull, bruised feeling and aching on attempting to rise. It is more suitable to the chronic forms of the lumbago. The backache of Rhus is better from pressure, but worse in bed. The Rhus tox patient wants to lie on something hard. Bending backward relieves pains. Pain between shoulders on swallowing. Stiffness of the nape of neck. Numbness and formication, after overwork and exposure.

BRYONIA: Painful stiffness in nape of neck. Stitches and stiffness in small of back. Backache from sudden changes of weather and from hard water. Every spot is painful on pressure. Bryonia suits lumbago of a quiet type, with great aggravation on moving. The general character of pain here produced is a stitching; tearing worse by motion, better by rest. Bryonia affects especially the constitution of a robust, firm fibre and dark complexion, with tendency to leanness and irritability. It prefers the right side, the evening and the open air.

NUX VOMICA: Another remedy in backache, especially if referable to spinal affections, is Nux vomica. It is in the lumber region, is worse at night when lying in bed, of a drawing, lacerating or bruised character, with perhaps sudden stitches in the back, and characteristic is that the patient must sit up in bed to turn over. It has also a morning backache and the longer the patient lies in bed the more the back aches. The backache brought on by sexual excesses should lead to the consideration of both Nux and Staphysgaria. Burning in spine; worse 3 to 4 a.m. cervico brachial neuralgia; worse touch. Must sit up in order to turn up in bed. Bruised pain below the scapular, sitting is painful. Nux patients are easily chilled, avoid open air. Nux is preeminently the remedy for many of the conditions incident to modern life. The typical nux patient is rather thin, quick, active, nervous and irritable.

SEPIA: It is frequently indicated in the backache, which is due to uterine diseases. There is general weakness in the small of back when walking and is worse while sitting. Sudden pain in the back as if struck by a hammer relieved by pressing back upon something hard. Coldness between shoulders. All pains are from below upwards. Tubercular patients with chronic hepatic troubles and uterine reflexes. Feels cold even in a warm room. Pain extends down to back, chills easily. Weakness yellow complexion, bearing down sensation especially in women.

CIMICIFUGA: It has violent aching in back in women, dependent on uterine complaints, especially in rheumatic subjects. Spine very sensitive especially upper part. Stiffness and contraction in neck and back. Intercoastal rheumatism. Rheumatic pains in the muscles of back and neck. Pain in lumbar and sacral region, down thighs and through hips. Crick in back. Pain like electric shock here and there. "It lessens the frequency and force of the pulse, soothes pain and allays irritability."

□□□

CHAPTER 33

Low Blood Pressure

Low blood pressure or hypotension is far less common than hypertension or high blood pressure. Sometimes the pressure falls rapidly because of hemorrhage or loss of blood. Low blood pressure may also come on gradually because of slow bleeding in the gastrointestinal tract or through the kidneys or bladder.

Any lack of normal protein in the diet may also lower the pressure because of malnutrition or actual starvation or because of some endocrine disturbance, such as hypothyroidism. In rare cases an islet cell tumor may form in the pancreas producing an excessive amount of insulin and lowering the blood sugar level. Such patients always tend to feel tired and worn out.

Emotional problems are a far more frequent cause of low blood pressure. For instance, some people will fall into a dead faint on hearing bad news. This shock like state is probably brought on by temporary disturbance in the vasomotor system, causing the patient to collapse. To a lesser degree, prolonged disappointment and frustration may also result in a subnormal blood pressure. Relieving the chronic stress of mind may be all that is needed to bring the blood pressure back to normal. One should also add a little more protein to the diet, and be sure to take sufficient rest and exercise.

Homoeopathic treatment for low blood pressure is given below:

Homoeopathic Medicines

GELSEMIUM : General weakness. Dizziness, drowsiness, dullness and trembling. Slow pulse tired feeling, mental apathy. Muscular weakness. Complete relaxation and prostration. Lack of muscular coordination. General depression from heat of sun. Cold and dampness brings on many complaints. Desire to be quite to be left alone. Delirious on falling to sleep. Bad effects from fright, fear, exciting news. Vertigo, spreading from occiput. Heaviness of head. Dull, heavy pain with heaviness of eyelids; bruised sensation, better compression and lying with head high. Headache proceeded by blindness; better by profuse urination. A feeling as f it was necessary to keep in motion, or else heart's action would cease. Palpitation of the heart.

CHINCHONA OFFICINALIS : Debility from exhausting discharges, from loss of vital fluids. Sensation as if brain were balancing to and fro, and striking against skull, receiving great pain. Intense throbbing of head and carotids. Spasmodic headache in vertex, with subsequent pain, as if bruised in sides of head. Face is flushed due to loss of vital fluids. Relieved from pressure and in warm room. Pain is worse in open air, from temple to temple. Blue color around eyes. Irregular with weak rapid beats followed by strong hard beats. Suffocative attacks, syncope, anaemia and dropsy. Pain in limbs and joints as if sprained. Great debility, trembling, with numb sensation. Aversion to exercise; sensitive to touch. Weariness of joints; worse mornings and when sitting.

PULSATILLA : The disposition and mental state are the chief guiding symptoms of this remedy. It is especially suited to mild, gentle, yielding females. Sad, crying readily; weeps when talking. The patient seeks the open air; always feel better there, even though the patient is chilly. Patient is timid and irresolute. Fears in evening to be alone. Likes sympathy. Easily discouraged. Highly emotional. Given to extremes of pleasure and pain. Morbid dread of the opposite sex.

SEPIA : Weakness, yellow complexion, bearing down sensation are the most important guiding symptoms of this remedy. Hot flushes at menopause with weakness and perspiration. Easy fainting. Feels cold even in warm room. Aversion to occupation, to family. Weeps when telling symptoms. Anxious towards evening. Vertigo with sensation of something rolling round the head. Stinging pain from within outward and upward mostly left, or in forehead, with nausea, vomiting; worse indoors and when lying on painful side. Jerking of head backwards and forwards. Face is yellowish in appearance.

ARSENIC ALB : Debility, exhaustion and restlessness with nightly aggravation are the leading indications for this remedy. Great exhaustion after the slight exertion. Burning pains. Unquenchable thirst for small quantities of water at small intervals. The patient has great deal of anguish and restlessness; he cannot lie down for fear of suffocation. There is anxiety and general sweat, and if the patient drowses off he is awakened with burning pain and soreness in the chest. Headache relieved by cold other symptoms worse. Head is in constant motion. Face is swollen, pale, yellow, cachetic, sunken cold and covered with sweat. Palpitation, pain, dsypnoea, faintness. Pulse more rapid in morning. Dilatation. Cyanosis. Angina pectoris with pain in neck and occiput. Great dsypnoea, attacks of suffocation at night on lying down and particularly after midnight.

DIGITALIS : It is known chiefly for its action on heart. The pulse is slow, but primarily strong, there is great weakness of the cardiac tissue and secondarily the pulse becomes weak. Extra exertion increased its rapidity but decreases its force, so that the quick pulse becomes irregular and intermittent. The heart feels as if the blood stood still. There is weakness and numbness of the left arm, and often blueness of the surface of the body, or cyanosis. The patient feels that the heart will stop beating if he should make any motion. This uneasy feeling about the chest rarely amounts to real pain. The digitalis patient has a doughy look to the skin; there is often a sick feeling at the stomach after eating. Disturbed sleep, apprehensive, deep, sighing, slow respiration, dry cough, suffocative spells. It is also indicated in dropsical constitution dependent on heart trouble, swelling of feet and ankles, anasarca, cardiac dropsy associated with slow pulse, urine suppressed or scanty. Inflammation of the heart muscles coming slowly and in sudden cases of myocarditis or endocarditis.

CARBO VEG : Lack of vitality, the coldness and weakness, the extreme exhaustion is prominent symptoms. Cannot bear tight clothing around waist and abdomen. Crampy pains forcing the patient to bend double. The patient wants to be fanned. It is useful remedy especially for the effects of overeating, high living or from eating tainted meats, where digestion being slow, the food putrefies before it digests. There is great craving for salt and other things, which makes him sick. The typical carbo patient is sluggish, fat and lazy and has a tendency to chronicity in his complaints. Blood seems to stagnate in the capillaries, causing blueness, coldness and ecchymosis. Vital power is decreased from loss of fluids. The patient may be almost lifeless. The patient faints easily, is worn out, and must have fresh air. Patient seems to be too weak. Indicated for persons who have never fully recovered from the effects of some previous illness. Sense of weight as in the head, eyes and eyelids. Vertigo with nausea and tinnitus.

❑❑❑

CHAPTER 34

Migraine

A neurotic headache, usually reflex in origin and paroxysmal in character.

The causes are many and varying in kind, making both the diagnosis and treatment the most difficult the general practioner encounters,

Migraine is clearly a hereditary condition, and the inheritance is passed down through the females rather than the males. Nervous abnormalities of the female generative organs are the most frequent of the exciting causes. Eye strain; shock; grief; worry; gastro-intestinal irregularities; mental emotions, i.e., anger, fear, love, jealously and remorse may cause migraine at one time and hysteria at another.

Many patients have lived, to suffer from the disease, for fifty years. On the other hand, many are permanently cured. The time needed to complete the cure will depend upon your ability to determine the tissue or organ, which is the cause of the disease, and the faithfulness with which the patient will follow directions.

Next to epilepsy, no disease so frequently presents premonitory symptoms as Hemicrania. These may be blurring of visions, flashes of light, balls of fire, etc.; chilliness; flashes of heat; dizziness; depression or excitation; confusion of ideas; numbness, etc. then comes the pain which is usually one sided, and may be any or all sensations, sharp or dull, continuous or intermittent, etc. There may or may not be tenderness of the affected part.

The face may be deathly pale or scarlet red; the veins of the affected side are distended; there are nausea and vomiting in the majority of cases, in some of which the pains are relieved by the vomiting, others are not; some are relieved by a good night's rest, while others are always worse after sleep. The average duration of an attack is about twenty-four hours, but suffer as long as seventy-two hours.

Homoeopathic Medicines

SCUTELLARIA: Since the students at Iowa University proved this remedy, I have relieved more patients of nervous sick headache with it than with any other remedy. The make up and use of this remedy are as follows: An intelligent, ambitious, highly neurotic, active woman, usually a leader in her club, church or society, with weak resisting powers. After attending a church or club function or theater party, she will come home excited, will go to bed and lie awake, living over again all she has heard and seen. There will be little or no sleep at night. The next day she will have a severe headache, aggravated by every noise, odor, or by light, which headache can only be relieved by a night's rest i.e., sleep. With the headache will be frequent urination, the amount of urine being scanty. This patient can be taught to take five drops of a good tincture of Scutellaria before going to bed, after a day's excitement and by so doing secure a good night's rest and thus avoid the attack the day afterwards. Sometimes a patient may require the second dose of five drops. If so, it can be repeated one hour after the first. Should you be called the day after, when the headache has appeared, give five drops every hour for three doses, after that every two hours.

IGNATIA: Is the great hysterical remedy. The form of headache known as "clovus" is peculiar to Ignatia. There are sharp piercing pains in the side of the head. The cause of the headache is usually grief, or some real or imaginary insult. The accompanying symptoms are: Frequent desire to urinate, the urine may be very profuse or scanty. The odor of the urine is pungent. The modalities of Ignatia are very prominent in this condition, especially that of a congestive headache relieved by hanging the head low. Give five drops of the 30th every half hour.

BELLADONA: This is the remedy for the young, plethoric, usually healthy, patient. The cause is some disturbance of the circulatory system. The headache is violent, pounding, throbbing, relieved by cold applications or having the head high. The face is flushed, the pulse full and bounding. Vertigo with falling to left side or backwards. Sensitive to least contact. Much throbbing and heat. Headache from suppressed catarrhal flow. Pain worse light, noise, jar, lying down and in afternoon; better by pressure and semi erect posture. Headache worse on right side and when lying down; ill effects, colds, etc. from having hair cut. Give the 30th. Five drops every half hour.

FERRUM PHOS: Greatly resembles Belladonna in its head symptoms. It has rush of blood to the head, throbbing and beating; also relief from cold applications. But the make up of the patient and the cause are different. Ferrum phos. is anemic, never plethoric. The causes are undue excitement and heat of the sun. Ill effects of sun heat. Throbbing sensation.

CHAMOMILLA : It has a throbbing beating headache in one-half of the brain from the following causes: the excessive use of morphine or coffee. It is the best remedy to restore the nervous tone, which the prolonged use of any of the preparations of opium has lowered or destroyed, strong emotions, especially anger; reflex irritations from the female genital organs. The head is hot and sweaty on the affected side. The face is also red and hot on the same side, but not on the other.

CIMICIFUGA : It has the feeling as if the brain were too large, a sensation as if the skull were opening and shutting, also shooting, throbbing pains. Cimicifuga also has sleeplessness because of the pain. Ease the pain and the patient will sleep. These patients nearly always suffer just before the menses. Many have a history of chorea or rheumatism. Mental depression and fear are leading symptoms.

IRIS VER : It cures a periodical, nervous, sick headache, which comes on after the patient relaxes from a mental strain. With school teachers to come every Saturday or Sunday; with preachers Monday etc. The above is the leading indication. The second most important symptoms is that the headache always begin with a blurring of vision. The Iris patient usually vomits a bitter, bilious substances and the vomiting gives relief to the pains of the head. In addition to the nerves, the liver and pancreas are often involved.

KALI BICH. : It produces a sick headache with a group of symptoms which is exact counterpart of those of Iris, except that the cause is catarrhal, catarrh of the sinuses or of the digestive tract. Vertigo with nausea when rising from seat. Headache over eyebrows, preceded by blurred vision. Aching and fullness in glabella. Frontal pains; usually over one eye. Bones and scalp feel sore.

SANGUINARIA: It is complementary to Spigelia in that it is a right-sided headache. It is also sun headache, which Sanguinaria cures, resembling Glonine and Ferrum Phos. The veins of the affected side of the head are greatly distended. There is burning in the stomach, nausea and vomiting. Vomiting always relieves the headache. Periodical sick headache begins in the occiput, spreads upwards, and settles over eyes, especially right. Pain better by lying down and sleep. Headache return at climacteric; every seventh day. Pain in the back of head "like a flash of lightning."

GELSEMIUM : It cures a headache, which is preceded by blurring of vision or even blindness. The head feels dull, full, and heavy. Passive congestion and heat of the sun are the two leading causes. The face is red, eyes suffused, pulse full but soft. The scalp is sore. The headache is relieved by profuse micturition. Vertigo spreading from occiput. Heaviness of head; band feeling around and occipital headache. Dull, heavy ache, with heaviness of eyelids; bruised sensation; better compression and lying with head high. Pain in temple, extending into ear and wing of nose, chin. Headache with muscular soreness of neck and shoulders.

CHAPTER 35

Mumps

It is an acute specific infection of the salivary glands especially of the parotids sometimes submandibular and sublingual glands also; occasionally the latter glands are affected first.

The most affected are the children or young adults of both sexes often living in a school or a barrack and the disease spreads rapidly from one person to another in close contact by droplets. This virus reaches the salivary glands by bloody or lymphatic because mumps is a systemic disease and may cause in addition, inflammation of the meninges, brain, pancreas and the gonads. The disease is more prevalent in winter and spring months. The incubation period is about 3 weeks.

The affected parotid glands and the surrounding tissues become hyperaemic and oedematous, the acinar cells disintegrate with round cell infiltration but later on, heal completely without any scarring.

Testes when involved have much oedema, perivascular infiltration with lymphocytes, localized haemorrhage, destruction of the germinal epithelia and blocking of the tubules with cellular debris. Only certain localized areas are affected, other parts remain unaffected.

The disease often starts insidiously with swelling of one parotid gland; the other being involved a day or two after. These become markedly tense and tender but the skin is not involved. The inflammation often spreads to sub maxillary and sublingual glands, the maximum being reached in three days. Mainly the interstitial and the periglandular tissues are involved and the swelling slowly subsides without suppuration. Sometimes relapses may occur after an interval of a few days, the parotids being inflamed again.

The temperature rises to 101°F. or more and continues for 3 to 4 days. During the period, the jaws are stiff and mastication is painful and difficult; salivation is sometimes marked. Pulse is usually slow. Blood shows slight initial leucopenia followed by marked lymphocytosis. The urine shows slight albuminuria. The serum amylase is increased in most patients in the first 3 to 4 days. Spleen may be just palpable.

Diagnosis is made from I) the prevalence of a localized epidemic: parotitis is nonsuppurating and bilateral ii) Complication of orchitis and iii) usually complete recovery.

a) Orchitis usually unilateral is especially marked in young adults: often starts form the 6th to 10th day of the disease when the parotid swelling has just commenced subsiding, with pain in the testis and a higher rise of temperature, less commonly, with severe constitutional disturbances. The inflammation may extend to the scrotum and spermatic cord and even to the inguinal glands. In most cases, the affection is unilateral and rarely bilateral. The inflammation often subsides in a week leaving no functional deficiency but sometimes leads to atrophy of the testicles.

b) In females, oophoritis is sometimes seen with inflammation of the vulva and mammae. Pregnant women may abort.

c) Rare complications are arthritis, bronchitis, pericarditis myocarditis and nephritis.

Homoeopathic medicines are available for mumps and their complications:

Homoeopathic Medicines

BELLADONNA: This is the most important remedy, corresponding to vascular engorgement, fever and nervous irritability. The glands are swollen, hot and red and sensitive to pressure, worse on right side. The pains are flying and lancinating and extend to the ear. It is also useful when the swelling suddenly subsides and is followed by throbbing headache and delirium. The headache is violent, pounding, throbbing, relieved by cold applications or having the head high. The face is flushed, the pulse full and bounding. Vertigo with falling to left side or backwards. Sensitive to least contact. Much throbbing and heat. Headache from suppressed catarrhal flow. Pain worse light, noise, jar, lying down and in afternoon; better by pressure and semi erect posture. The patient is excitable, worries over small things, is violent in emotions, the pulse is full, rapid, bounding, there is throbbing in the carotids, the temperature of the skin is increased, the skin may be moist or dry, the eyeballs are prominent, pain deep in the eyeballs, the pupils dilated, the mucous membrane dry, the lids stiff, swollen and dry.

RHUS TOX : It is indicated for the dark red swellings, with tendency to erysipelatous inflammation and typhoid conditions. There is much aching in the limbs, the patient is restless and the symptoms are worse at night. It is the best remedy in secondary parotitis. The left side is more frequently affected. Aggravation from rest and over exertion and amelioration from change of position and heat are the ranking modalities of Rhustox. Sticking pain on swallowing. Postoperative complications. Ailments from strains, over lifting, get wet while perspiring. Septic conditions. Want of appetite for any kind of food, with unquenchable thirst. Bitter taste. Great thirst, with dry mouth and throat.

MERCURIUS : This is one of the best remedies for mumps, as it has a specific action on the salivary glands. There is slight fever and it is useful in the later stages. The special symptoms are tenderness, salivation, offensive breath and threatening suppuration. It has great dryness and soreness of the throat, the patient is obliged to swallow constantly and there is much soreness and swelling of the glands externally. The throat is raw and burning and also red and swollen.. An offensive breathe from the mouth is a guiding symptom. Bluish red swelling. Constant desire to swallow. Putrid sore throat; worse right side. Ulcers and inflammation appearing at every change of weather. Stitches into ear on swallowing. Quinsy with difficult swallowing after pus has formed. Sore, raw, smarting, burning throat. Complete loss of voice. Burning in throat, as from hot vapor ascending.

PULSATILLA : Especially useful in orchitis and mammary complications. The tongue is thickly coated, the mouth is dry and the pains are worse evenings and after lying down. For metastasis to the ovaries Pulsatilla may be the remedy. The patient seeks the open air; always feel better there, even though he is chilly. It is preeminently a female remedy, especially for mild, gentle, yielding disposition. Sad, crying readily, weeps when talking; changeable; contradictory. Mucous membranes are all affected. Prosopalgia towards evening till midnight; chilly with pain.

BARYTA CARBONICA : Its use especially when the trouble is in the parenchyma of the glands and suppuration follows its use. It removes the predisposition to attack Belladonna is more superficial and Apis has oedema. It is useful where every cold settles in the tonsils. Especially in children who have chronic enlargement of those glands. The main use of Baryta has been, however in chronic enlargement of the tonsils. In a tendency to tonsillitis to scrofulous children with enlargement of other glands it will be found useful. Belladonna seems to have an affinity for right side. Children are backward and bashful requiring Baryta.

□□□

CHAPTER 36

Myocarditis - Acute & Chronic

An inflammation of the muscular substance of the heart. The condition may be acute or chronic. Acute myocarditis may be sub-divided into three varieties:

1. Acute Parenchyma.
2. Acute Diffuse Interstitial.
3. Acute Circumscribed.

In the first of three classes, there is a glandular degeneration of the muscular fibres of the parenchyma of the heart and an increase in the number of their nuclei. Severe cases of this class often terminate in fatty degeneration.

In the second class, we have round-cell infiltration of connective tissue of the myocardium.

In the third class, there is necrosis of tissue with abscess. These abscesses are usually multiple, vary greatly in number and when they rupture discharge into the different cardiac chambers or into the pericardium. As a result of the ruptured abscess we may have emboli of various viscera, aneurisms of the heart wall, mitrial or tricuspid insufficiency, etc. on the other hand the abscess may become encysted and remain so or undergo a caseous and calcareous process.

Myocarditis may be the result of rheumatic or paricarditis, i.e., following them; or it may be result of rheumatism without the pericardium being involved. Infectious processes of acute specific fevers. Infectious emboli from septicemia or pyemic processes.

The pulse is rapid, weak, compressible, and arithmetic, palpitation of the heart; pallor; syncope; vomiting; heart action weak, irregular and feeble; systolic blood pressure low 100 to 75; frequent murmurs in the myocardium. In the more advanced stages the regurgitant murmur of the tricuspid valves and the venous pulse may be added to the list of symptoms.

Chronic Myocarditis

Inflammation of the interstitial connective tissue of the heart gradually developing into duration. These indurated spots are gray, grayish-white or grayish-yellow in colour. The changed spots are most frequently found in certain sections of the muscular structures, of the left ventricular wall, of the sputum, of the papillary muscles; but the induration may be diffuse. The spots vary in size from a spec to two inches. We often find narrowing of the pulmonary and aortic orifices. Dilatation of the ventricles and compensating hypertrophy coronaries may be affected, causing thrombosis and anemic infarcts. Microscopically we find hyperplasia of the inter- fibrillar connective tissue caused by development of new fibrinous tissue. Fatty degeneration and atrophy of the muscle fibers occasionally occur.

In these days, a primary local focus in the teeth, tonsils, gall bladder or other organs is credited with being the cause of many cases; alcohol and tobacco have been arraigned and found guilty; workers in or with lead, phosphorus, arsenic and corrosive substances have suffered from the disease, malaria, syphilis and diabetes have all been etiological factor

Many patients die of some other disease and the post mortem reveals the fact that the disease existed without the patient or his physician being aware of it. The cerebral symptoms are syncope, mental weakness also occasionally pseudo- apoplectic attacks; the left ventricle is enlarged, giving weakness and muffling of the heart sounds; the pulmonary second sound of the heart is accentuated and in some cases reduplicated; both the force and frequency of the heart are irregular. When there is dilatation an apical, systolic murmur and a gallop rhythm of the heart occur. When the papillary muscles and the chordae tendinea are contracted we have mitrial incompetence with the usual murmur during compensation.

Treatment for myocarditis in homoeopathy is given as under:

Homoeopathic Medicines

BRYONIA : It has a marked elective affinity for muscular tissues as well as serous tissue. Patient has aggravation from motion. Patient is chilly. Bryonia affects especially the constitution of a robust, firm fibre and dark complexion, with tendency to leanness and irritability. It prefers the right side, the evening and the open air. Lying on the right or painful side relieves the pains in the chest, besides being worse by motion and breathing,, because that lessens the motion of that side. It corresponds to first and second stage of pericarditis when of rheumatic origin and if pleuritic symptoms are present. There is intense fever, frontal or occipital headache and acute stitching pains, which are aggravated by movement and the friction murmur, is always present. Cramp in the region of heart, aggravated by walking, rising one self or using the slightest exertion even raising the arm. Heart beats violently and rapidly.

DIGITALIS : It is known chiefly for its action on heart. The pulse is slow, but primarily strong, there is great weakness of the cardiac tissue and secondarily the pulse becomes weak. Extra exertion increased its rapidity but decreases its force, so that the quick pulse becomes irregular and intermittent. The heart feels as if the blood stood still. There is weakness and numbness of the left arm, and often blueness of the surface of the body, or cyanosis. The patient feels that the heart will stop beating if he should make any motion. This uneasy feeling about the chest rarely amounts to real pain. The digitalis patient has a doughy look to the skin; there is often a sick feeling at the stomach after eating. Disturbed sleep, apprehensive, deep, sighing, slow respiration, dry cough, suffocative spells. It is also indicated in dropsical constitution dependent on heart trouble, swelling of feet and ankles, anasarca, cardiac dropsy associated with slow pulse, urine suppressed or scanty. Inflammation of the heart muscles coming slowly and in sudden cases of myocarditis or endocarditis.

CACTUS : It is one of the heart remedies. Its most important symptom that the "Sensation as if the heart were grasped with an iron band," which clutches and relaxes alternately is always present. There is pain in the chest shooting into the left arm, oedema and a quick, throbbing, tense, hard pulse, which may or may not intermit. Carditis and pericarditis may call for this remedy. It controls the inflammatory conditions and strengthens the heart's contractions. There is great irritation of the cardiac nerves and angina pectoris is also present. It is a remedy adapted to hypertrophy of the heart in young people. It is also very useful in intense palpitation and fluttering sensation about the heart. Difficult breathing, suffocating, fainting, violent palpitation and inability to lie down are important symptoms indicating for this remedy.

KALMIA : It is the remedy for cardiac hypertrophy, especially after rheumatism. Numbness of the left arm. There is much pain and anguish about the heart, some dsypnoea, palpitation and pressure from the epigastrium towards the heart. The heart is irregular and intermits every third or fourth beat. There are shooting pains through the chest to the scapula. Kalmia is an excellent remedy for cardiac troubles when they have been caused by the suppression of rheumatism by external applications. The pulse is slow. The sharp pains taking away the breath calls for this remedy.

SPIGELIA : It is the remedy for the painful affections about the heart. There are sharp pains shooting from the heart to the back, and radiating from the heart down the arm, over the chest, and down the spine. There is palpitation worse from any movement of the arm or body. There is a purring sensation felt over the cardiac region when placing the hand thereon. The pulse is intermittent, not synchronous with the heartbeat, and the slightest motion of the arm or hands makes the patient worse. Heart symptoms accompany neuralgia. Irregular and tumultuous action of the heart. At times the heartbeat is audible. This remedy will often cure rheumatic endocarditis. It has the most beneficial action in the angina pectoris. It corresponds well to chronic affections of the heart, particularly valvular disease and hypertrophy.

CHAPTER 37

Obesity

It is very important to watch weight, not allowing oneself to become too thin or too fat, but trying to remain neat ideal. Most youngsters in their teens, if they are healthy and active, are fairly close to the ideal weight for their size and age. Changes often come in the late twenties, reducing a person's physical fitness. Sluggish habits begin to develop as the individual loses his skill in running, swimming or healthy activities.

When greater quantities of energy (in the form of food) enter the body than are expended, the body weight increases. Therefore, obesity is caused by excess energy input over energy output. In other words, extra weight is due to extra eating. For each 9.3 Calories of excess energy that enters the body, one gram of fat is stored.

Excess energy input occurs only during the development phase of obesity. Once a person has become obese, all that is required to remain obese so that the energy input equals the energy output. For a person to reduce in weight, the input must be less than the output. People with large bones and well-developed muscles may seem somewhat overweigh compared with those of lighter build. But actually the lighter person may carry around more fat. His muscles may be weak and underdeveloped.

How many calories do one need per day. It all depends on a number of things, such as the kind of work one do, age, body build and how active one is. A hard working labourer may require 5,000 calories per day. His wife, who is busy around the house all day, may need 2500 calories. But an office secretary may require only 1800 calories a day. It all depends on how active one is.

Effect of muscular activity on energy output

About one third of the energy used each day by the normal person goes into muscular activity, and in the laborer, as much as two third or occasionally three fourth is used. Because muscular activity is by far the most important means by which energy is expended in the body, it is frequently said that obesity in the otherwise normal person results from too high a ratio of food intake to daily exercise.

Different causes of obesity

1. *Abnormal feeding regulation:* The rate of feeding is normally regulated in proportion to the energy stores in the body. When these stores exceed a normal level for a normal person, feeding is automatically reduced to prevent over storage.
2. *Psychogenic obesity:* A large number of obesity results from psychogenic factors. The most important psychogenic factor contributing to obesity so the prevalent idea that healthy eating habits require three meals a day and each meal must be filling. May young children are forced into this habit by their parents. Some people also gain weight during or after stressful situations, such as the death of a parent, a severe illness, or even mental depression. Some people think that eating as a means of relieving tension.
3. *Neurogenic abnormalities as a cause of obesity:* Lesions in the ventromedial nuclei of the hypothalamus cause an animal to eat excessively and become obese. Such lesions also cause excess insulin production, which in turn increases fat deposition. In addition, many people with hypophysial tumours that develops on the hypothalamus result in progressive obesity.
4. *Genetic factors in the obesity:* Obesity definitely runs in families. Furthermore, identical twins usually maintain weight levels within 2 ponds of each other throughout life if they live under similar conditions, or within 5 pounds of each other if their conditions of life differ markedly.
5. *Childhood over nutrition as a possible cause:* The rate of formation of new fat cells is especially rapid in the first few years of life, and the greater the rate of fat storage, the greater also becomes the number of fat cells. In obese children, the number of fat cells is often as much as three times that in normal children. Therefore it has been observed that over nutrition of children especially in infancy and to a lesser extent during the later years of childhood can lead to a lifetime of obesity.

How to lose weight

Dieting is not new to most people who are overweight. They have all tried this many times before. The only solution is a completely new pattern of life, such as given below:

1. *Take smaller quantities of food:* A balanced diet should be taken. Include reasonable amounts of potatoes and also take whole grain cereals in you diet.
2. *Stop nibbling between meals:* Train yourself to get along less food. You will enjoy living on a reduced diet.
3. *Be careful about " left - over:* Mostly house wives put on weight because they hate to see food wasted. It is better to prepare less food and avoid the problem of " left - over".
4. *Sensible exercise:* Exercise taken everyday. Walking is the best exercise. Burn up unwanted calories by putting large leg muscles to work.
5. *Avoid rich deserts:* Excess sugar and fat is high in calories but low in food value. Push yourself away from the table is the best exercise. Although you are still hungry. Never take Ice- cream, pastry, rich cakes and sweets.
6. Regular eating is the most important. Meals should be well prepared, smaller and attractively arranged on the table. Enjoy your meals.
7. *Don't go hungry for long:* Eating regularly but sparingly the best way to lose weight.
8. *Be sure to have a good & light breakfast :* Breakfast will carry you through the day.
9. *Freely use these foods :* Green leafy vegetables, tomatoes and carrots. They are low in calories, but high in vitamins and minerals and have real food value.

Homoeopathic Medicines

CALCAREA CARB : It is indicated for the children who grow fat, are large belied, with large head, pale skin, chalky look. Children crave eggs and eat dirt and other indigestible things. Its chief action is on the vegetative sphere. Increased local and general perspiration. Calcarea patient is fat, fair, flabby and perspiring. Swollen abdomen. Cannot tolerate tight clothing around the waist. Patient is worse from exertion, mental or physical. Anxiety with palpitation. Aversion to work or exertion. Sense of weight on top of head. Loss of appetite when overworked. Cramps in stomach; worse pressure, cold water. Ravenous hunger. Swelling over pit of stomach, like a saucer turned bottom up. Pain in epigastric region to touch. Thirst, longing for cold drinks. Swelling of tonsils and sub maxillary glands.

ARSENIC ALB: It is a profoundly acting remedy on every organ and tissues. Debility, exhaustion and restlessness with nightly aggravation are the leading indications for this remedy. Great exhaustion after the slight exertion. Burning pains. Unquenchable thirst for small quantities of water at small intervals. Injurious effects of fruits especially juicy fruits. Anxiety in pit of stomach. Craves acid and coffee. Long lasting eructation. Gastralgia from slightest food or drink. Everything swallowed seemed to lodge in the oesophagus which seems as if closed and nothing would pass. Liver and spleen enlarged and painful. Craves milk.

❏❏❏

CHAPTER 38

Piles

Haemorrhoids or piles are due to swelling or enlargement of the veins that supply the rectal outlet of the body. Localized inflammation and bleeding, and also thrombosis in many cases often complicate this painful condition. People who suffer from constipation and other bowel disorders are more likely to develop haemorrhoids. Piles are also more common in pregnancy, and in conditions affecting the liver and upper bowel.

There are two types of haemorrhoids:

1) External haemorrhoids

2) Internal haemorrhoids.

External haemorrhoids are more common, for they lie outside the anorectal junction.

Internal hemorrhoids are soft and dark coloured, and usually irregular in shape. When very large, they may protrude through the anus. Straining at the stool may bring them down. This may be followed by strangulation of the hemorrhoids with severe pain.

These may be from:

a) Portal stasis

b) Pelvic diseases as frequent pregnancies, uterine displacement and new pelvic growth.

c) Habitual constipation especially of persons taking spicy foods and alcohol.

Haemorrhoids are the most common cause of the rectal bleeding. The blood is bright red and may be noted on the toilet paper, and also covering the surface of the stool or dripping into the toilet bowl after the stool is passed. However because cancer of the rectum may possibly also be present, a thorough examination should be done in all cases of haemorrhoids.

Small haemorrhoids that cause only slight bleeding may not require any treatment. The patient should take at least six to eight glasses of water a day. The diet should be rich in fruits and vegetables. He should avoid straining at stool. Pruritis ani may be associated.

Homoeopathic Medicines

AESCULUS: This remedy is especially suitable to the form of haemorrhoids from portal congestion, abdominal plethora. They may or may not bleed, but there is a feeling in the rectum as of splinters or sticks. Other indicating symptoms are aching in the lumber region, protruding purple piles with severe pains in the sacrum and small of the back and fullness in the region of the liver. Dryness, burning and itching are good indications. Haemorrhoids from chronic constipation may be cured with this medicine. Anus raw and sore. Much pain after stool, with prolapse. Large, dry and hard stools. Mucous membrane seems swollen and obstructs the passage. Burning in anus with chills up and down back. Haemorrhoids, with sharp shooting pains up the back, blind and bleeding.

COLLINSONIA : Obstinate cases of haemorrhoids, which bleed almost incessantly. It is of special use in females with inertia of the rectum and a congestive tendency to the pelvic organs. It suits pregnant women who suffer from piles, and pruritis may be marked. The indicating symptoms are chiefly a sensation of sticks in the rectum, with constipation from inertia of the lower bowel. It is especially applicable to heart pains resulting from a suppression of a habitual haemorrhoidal flow. Vascular engorgement of rectum. Aching in anus and hypogastrium. Alternate constipation and diarrhoea and great flatulence. Itching of anus. Pain on sitting down. Dry faeces.

NUX VOMICA: If the haemorrhoids be large and blind, with a burning, stinging and constricted feeling in the rectum and a bruised pain in the small of back, and especially occurs in persons of sedentary habits, or abuse of stimulants. Itching haemorrhoids keeping the patient awake at night' relieved by cold water, or bleeding piles with constant urging to stool, and a feeling as if the bowel would not empty itself. Constipation with frequent ineffectual urging, incomplete and unsatisfactory; feeling as if part remained unexpelled. Alternate constipation and diarrhoea- after abuse of purgatives. Scanty stool, with much urging. Renal colic extending to genitals, with dribbling urine. Bruised pain below the scapular, sitting is painful. Nux patients are easily chilled, avoid open air. Nux is preeminently the remedy for many of the conditions incident to modern life. The typical nux patient is rather thin, quick, active, nervous and irritable.

ALOES : This is also a most useful haemorrhoidal remedy. It is indicated when the piles protrude like a bunch of grapes, bleeding often and profusely, and are greatly relieved by the application of cold water. There is a very marked burning in the anus, the bowels as if scraped. There is tendency to diarrhoea, with uncertain felling in the lower bowel. Constant bearing down in rectum; bleeding sore and hot. Feeling of weakness and loss of power of sphincter ani. Sense of insecurity in rectum when passing flatus. Jelly like stools, with soreness in rectum after stool. Burning in anus and rectum. Constipation with heavy pressure in lower part of abdomen.

HAMMAMELIS : It is one of the best remedies in haemorrhoids. It has bleeding haemorrhoids and the flow of blood is quite copious and the great characteristic indication is excessive soreness. Anus feels sore and raw. Pulsation in rectum. Pain in spermatic cord, running into testis. Bearing down pain in back. Acts upon the coats of the veins causing relaxation with consequent engorgement. Passive venous haemorrhages from any part. Great weakness from loss of blood.

SULPHUR : This remedy corresponds to ailments producing haemorrhoids and to troubles resulting from piles, which have stopped bleeding, and as a result fullness in the head and uneasiness in the liver; constipation is present, a desire for stool and itching at anus. Itching and burning at anus. Redness around the anus. Haemorrhoids, oozing and belching. When carefully selected remedies fail to act, especially in acute diseases, it frequently arouses the reactionary powers of the organism. Very red lips and face, flushing easily. Often-great use in beginning the treatment of chronic cases and finishing the acute ones. Itching, burning of the skin, worse scratching and washing. The stools are hard, dark, dry and expelled with great straining the first effort to stool being extremely painful. There is apt to be much twitching and burning of the anus, the evacuations are often unsatisfactory and there is a sensation as if a part is left behind. Another characteristic of Sulphur is that diarrhoea alternates with constipation.

CHAPTER 39

Pneumonia

Pneumonia was once one of the most dreaded diseases known to man. It is no longer so. But pneumonia is still a serious disease. Germs causing pneumonia re of various types, such as streptococcus, staphylococcus, and pneumococcus varieties. Certain viruses are also responsible at times.

Pneumonia may be defined as an acute infectious disease of the lung, caused by the micrococcus lanceoaltus affecting principally the parenchyma.

The lesions are divided into the following stages:

1) Congestion or engorgement.

2) Consolidation

3) Resolution.

In the first stage the portion of the lung implicated gives us a dark red color, a harder feeling, yet less resilient than normal. On section, blood stained serum, and blood darker than normal appears.

On microscopic examination the alveolar epithelium is found swollen, the capillaries greatly distended and the air cells contain epithelial cells and a few leucocytes.

In the second stage we find the tissues resembling liver tissues, solid, airless and firm. The color is of mahogany, presenting a mottled appearance. No air is found in the tissue and its weight is greatly increased. The tissue cannot be inflated as in the first stage, but is extremely pliable and when broken down presents a finely granular aspect. In our postmortems of patients dying in this stage, we find that dry exudates formed ante mortem may soon become a grumous fascid fluid. The tissue at this stage rapidly sinking in the water. We find the pulmonary pleura of this stage covered with fibrin, and in many cases we have complication of pleurisy and the sac may contain a fluid.

In the third stage, the fibrinous exudate loses its color, appearing uniformly gray. At this stage we find fatty granular degeneration of the inflammatory exudates, which looses its granular character and becomes more friable, terminating in a grayish white, or yellowish white purulent liquid.

The predisposing causes are epidemic and endemic influences, climate, exposure, traumatism, age and sex; the exciting or specific cause is the diplococus.

Pneumonia begins with a chill or chilliness. The chill is usually more pronounced in the young. The chill is followed by a rapid rise of temperature, which often reaches 105 or 106. Convulsions often occur in children at this stage. As a rule sharp, lancinating, tearing, sticking pains are present. The more extensive the pleuritis accompanying the pneumonia, the more severe the pain. Cough is usually present, though in some cases cough is absent; when present it is at first dry and hacking, later the rust color sputum appears with the cough and still later the expectoration may be purulent or mucopurulent. There is usually present headache, malaise, hot skin, loss of appetite, flushed face, full hard pulse, hurried difficult breathing and constriction of the chest.

During the second stage there are some changes, the pain is usually less, the dsypnoea more marked, the pulse weaker, the expectoration more profuse and less adhesive, there is less motion of the chest and more dullness as no air enters the affected part of the lung.

During the stage of resolution all symptoms become less severe and there is general improvement, unless some complications set in or purulent in filtration takes place, in which case the pulse becomes more rapid, weaker and sometimes intermittent. The expectorations become more purulent; the patient becomes weaker, unable to expectorate the accumulated debris and the patient has asphyxia. Delirium occurs in some cases. It is usually an unfavorable symptom, especially if coming during the last stage with other typhoid symptom like dry tongue; sordes on the teeth, etc. and if the delirium is present it is of a low muttering type. Delirium coming with the high temperature of the first stage is not so dangerous.

Homoeopathic Medicines

ACONITE : It is the remedy in the first stage of the pneumonia, because it corresponds to the symptoms usually found in this stage. High fever proceeded by a distinct chill; the pulse is full, hard and tense; a history of exposure may also be taken into consideration; dry cold winds. The skin is hot and dry, without moisture upon it; there is a hard, dry, teasing and painful cough; some expectoration may be present, if so it is watery, serous and frothy, maybe blood tinged, but not thick. There is pain also with Aconite, which is poorly borne. There is great restlessness, tossing about, anxiety and fear of death. There is suddenness of onset of the symptoms and especially in young and plethoric persons who are full of life and vigour. Constant pressure in left chest; oppressed breathing on least motion. Cough, dry, short, hacking, worse at night and after midnight. Blood comes up with hawking.

VERATRUM VIRIDE : In violent congestions about the chest preceding pneumonia Veratrum viride may be the remedy, and thus it is seen that its use is more in the beginning of the disease, and especially where there is great arterial excitement, dyspnoea, chest oppression and stomach symptoms of nausea and vomiting; the engorgement is profound. There is high fever, violent action of the heart, the pulse is full, hard and rapid and the tongue has a red streak down the center. The air cells at the bottom of the lobes are filling up with frothy mucus. Sensation of a heavy load on chest. Pneumonia with faint feeling in stomach and violent congestion. Congestion of lungs. Difficult breathing. Especially adapted to full blooded, plethoric persons. Congestive stage and early manifestations of hepatization in pneumonia.

BRYONIA : It is the remedy for pneumonia. The fever continues but the skin is not as hot and the patient not as restless as in Aconite. The cough of Bryonia is looser and moister than that of Aconite, and there are usually sharp stitching pleuritic pains, the cough of Bryonia is also hard and dry at times and the sputum is scanty and rust coloured. There may be circumscribed redness of the cheeks, slight delirium and apathy, the tongue will most likely to be dry, and the patient will want to keep perfectly quiet. It is right-sided remedy and attacks the parenchyma of the lung, and is perhaps more strongly indicated in the croupous form of pneumonia. The patient dreads to cough and holds his breath to prevent it on account of the pain it causes; it seems as though the chest walls would fly to pieces. The pains in the chest, besides being worse by motion and breathing, a re relieved by lying on the right or painful side, because that lessens the motion of that side. Cough that hurts distant parts of the body calls for bryonia. In pneumonia complicated by pleurisy Bryonia is the remedy.

PHOSPHORUS: It is the "the great mogul of lobar pneumonia". It should be remembered that Phosphorus is not like Bryonia, the remedy when the lungs are completely hepatized, although it is one of the few drugs, which have been known to produce hapatisation. When bronchial symptoms are present it is the remedy. There is cough, with pain under sternum, a s if something were torn loose; there is pressure across the upper part of the chest and constriction of the larynx; there are mucous rales; labored breathing, sputa yellowish mucus, with blood streaks therein, or rust colored, as under Bryonia. When typhoid symptoms occur in the course of pneumonia then Phosphorus will be the remedy. There is also a sensation as if the chest were full of blood, which causes an oppression of breathing.

ANTIMONIUM TARTARICUM : This drug is especially indicated in pneumonia and pleuro- pneumonia at the stage of resolution. There are fine moist rales heard all over the hepatized portion of the lungs. With Antimonium tart there is great oppression of breathing, worse towards morning, compelling the patient to sit up to breathe. There are also sharp, stitching pains and high fever, perhaps it corresponds more to the catarrhal form than it does to the croupous form. There is one peculiar symptom, the patient feels sure that the next cough will raise the mucus, but it does not. When there is deficient reaction as in the aged or very young children, this remedy is particularly indicated. Oedema and impending paralysis of lungs. Bronchial tubes loaded with mucus. Cough excited by eating, with pain in chest and larynx. Dizziness with cough. Dsypnoea relieved by eructation. Cough and dyspnoea better by lying on right side.

□□□

CHAPTER **40**

Prostate Disorders

The testis is composed of up to 900-coiled seminiferous tubules, each averaging more than 0.5 meter long, in which the sperm are formed. The sperm than empty in to the epididymitis, another coiled tube about 6 meters long. The epididymis leads into the vas deferens, which enlarges in to the ampulla of the vas deferens immediately before the vas enters the body of the prostrate gland. A seminal vesicle, one located on each side of the prostrate, empties into the prostatic end of the ampulla, and the contents from both the ampulla and the seminal vesicle pass into an ejaculatory duct leading through the body of the prostrate gland to empty from the prostrate gland into the ejaculatory duct. Finally the urethra is the last connecting link from the testis to the exterior.

The prostrate gland secretes a thin, milky fluid that contains citrate ion, calcium, phosphate ion, a clotting enzyme, and a profibrinolysin. During emission, the capsule of the prostrate gland contracts simultaneously with the contractions of the vas deferens so that the thin, milky fluid of the prostrate glands adds further to the bulk of the semen. Slightly characteristic of the prostatic fluid may be quite important for successful fertilization of the ovum because the fluid of the vas deferens is relatively acidic owing to the presence of citric acid and metabolic end products of the sperm and consequently, helps to inhibit sperm fertility. The vaginal secretions of the female are acidic. Sperm do not become optimally motile until the pH of the surrounding fluids rises to about 6.5. Consequently, it is probable the prostatic fluid helps to neutralize the acidity of these other fluids after ejaculation and thus enhances the motility and fertility of the sperm.

The prostate gland remains relatively small throughout childhood and begins to grow at puberty under the stimulus of testosterone. This gland reaches an almost stationary size by the age of 20 years and remains at the size up to the age of 50 years. At that time in some men it begins to involutes, along with the decreased production of testosterone by the testes. A benign prostatic fibroadenoma frequently develops in the prostate in many older men and can cause urinary obstruction. This hypertrophy is not caused by testosterone.

Cancer of the prostate gland is a common cause of death, resulting in about 3% of all male deaths. Once cancer of the prostate gland does occur the cancerous cells are usually stimulated to more rapid growth by testosterone and are inhibited by removal of prostatic cancer that has already metastasized to almost all the bones of the body can be successfully treated for a few months to years by removal of the testes, by estrogen therapy, or by both. After this therapy the metastases usually diminish in size and the bones partially heal. This treatment does not stop the cancer but does slow it and sometimes greatly diminishes the severe bone pain.

Homoeopathy has a very good treatment for prostatic disorders. Some of the important useful homoeopathic medicines are given below:

Homoeopathic Medicines

SABAL SERRULATA: This medicine has been recommended for various prostatic troubles, but its use is only confined to acute cases of enlarged and inflamed prostate. The gland is hot, swollen and painful. It is also a very useful remedy in hypertrophy of the gland in old people. General and sexual debility. Its acts on membrano-prostatic portion of urethra. Iritis with prostatic trouble. Discharge of prostatic fluid. Wasting of testis and loss of sexual power. Coitus painful at the time of emission. Organs feel cold. Constant desire to pass urine at night. Enuresis; paresis of sphincter vesicae. Difficult urination. Cystitis with prostatic hypertrophy.

CONIUM : This remedy is useful in chronic hypertrophy of the prostate with difficulty in voiding urine, it stops and starts, and there is an accompanying catarrh of the bladder. It is also suitable remedy for the complaints of the old people. Debility, hypochondriasis, urinary troubles, weakened memory, sexual debility are some of the important symptoms pointing to this remedy. Great debility in the morning in bed. Acts on the glandular system, engorging and indurating it, altering its structure like scrofulous and cancerous conditions. Sexual desire is increased but power is decreased, sexual nervousness, with feeble erection. Effects of suppressed sexual appetite. Testicles hard and enlarged. Much difficulty in passing the urine. It flows and stops again. Interrupted discharge. Dribbling in old men.

THUJA : Frequent pressing to urinate with small discharge. Patient strains much. Stitches from rectum into bladder. Discharge of prostatic fluid in the morning on awaking. Inflammation of prepuce and glans; pain in penis. Chronic induration of testicles. Pain and burning felt near neck of bladder, with frequent and urgent desire to urinate. Prostatic enlargement. The main action of Thuja is on the skin and genitourinary organs producing conditions that corresponds with Hahnemann's sycotic dyscrasia whose chief manifestations is the formation of wart like excrescences upon mucous and cutaneous surfaces, fig warts and condylomata has a specific antibacterial action as in gonorrhoea and vaccination. Urethra swollen, inflamed. Urinary stream split and small. Sensation of trickling after urinating. Frequent micturition accompanying pains. Desire sudden and urgent, but cannot be controlled. Paralysis of sphincter vesicae.

DIGITALIS : Nightly emissions, with great weakness of genitals after coitus. Hydrocele; scrotum enlarged like a bladder. Gonorrhoea, balanitis with edema of prepuce. Dropsical swelling of the genitals. Enlarged prostate. Continued urging to urinate, urine in drops, dark, hot, burning with sharp cutting or throbbing pain at neck of bladder, as if a straw was being thrust back and forth; worse at night. Urethritis, phimosis, strangury. Full feeling after urination. Constriction and burning as if urethra was too small. The pulse is weak, irregular, intermittent, abnormally slow, and dropsy of external and internal parts. Prostration from slight exertion.

ARGENTUM NITRICUM : Symptoms of in coordination, loss of control and want of balance everywhere, mentally and physically are the great indications for this remedy. Impotency. Erection fails when coition is attempted. Cancer like ulcers. Coition painful. Urine passes unconsciously, day and night. Urethra inflamed, with pain, burning, itching, pain as from splinter. Urine scanty and dark. Emission of a few drops after having finished. Early stage of gonorrhoea; profuse discharge and terrible cutting pains; bloody urine. It is an irritant of mucous membranes, producing violent inflammation of the throat and a marked gastroenteritis.

GELSEMIUM : Spermatorrhoea, without erections. Genitals cold and relaxed. Scrotum continually sweating. Gonorrhoea, first stage; discharge scanty; tendency to corrode; little pain, but much heat; smarting at meatus. Urine profuse, clear, watery, with chilliness and tremulousness. Paralysis of bladder; flow intermittent. Retention of urine. The headache is relieved by profuse micturition. The patient is dull and weak, chills run up and down the back, with a watery, excoriating, or bland discharge from the nose and sneezing. General weakness. Dizziness, drowsiness, dullness and trembling. Slow pulse tired feeling, mental apathy. Muscular weakness. Complete relaxation and prostration. Lack of muscular coordination. General depression from heat of sun. Cold and dampness brings on many complaints. Desire to be quite to be left alone. Delirious on falling to sleep. Bad effects from fright, fear, exciting news.

□□□

CHAPTER 41

Psoriasis

This is characterized by formation of erythematous papules or patches with clear margins and covered with white scales, in different parts of the body without any constitutional disturbances.

It is more common among young adults of either sex and occasionally a family history is present. This has a seasonal prevalence often appearing in winter and clearing up in summer.

The course in chronic is very obstinate and tends to recur after an apparent cure. It disappears without leaving scars or pigmentation. It is not infectious.

The epithelial layer is thickened and intercappilary processes and papillae are elongated, the horny layer is defective and there is cellular infiltration between the horny cells and blood vessels.

The disease usually starts as a tiny erthymatous papule with thin scales on the top, which may not be visible to the naked eye, but on scraping the surface, dry silver white scales are demonstrated. As more silvery or miraculous scales are heaped up, it gradually enlarges centrifugally may be forming one continuous sheet. The size varies from that of pea to several inches. May be many, of the size of raindrops and bigger rings. Coming together form convulated figures. These may be in only localized patches involving the extensors or the flexures of the body.

The localized patches are usually on the tip of the elbows, over the patella; sometimes the lumbosacral region, calves, forearm and the scalp. The flexures are involved, these being in the axillae, sub mammary folds, umbilicus genitocrural folds and the intergluteal clefts. Sometimes the disease is more generalized and may be associated with constitutional disturbances. The nails are characteristically pitted or striated with thick masses of scales underneath. Slight itching may be present in some cases. General health is not impaired.

Homoeopathic Medicines

GRAPHITES : Our great remedy for all sorts of skin diseases. The symptoms calling for it are very clear; there are moist scabby eruptions on the scalp, face, bends of joints, between fingers and behind the ears. The corners of the mouth and eyes are cracked, bleeding and oozing a gluey, home-like, thick, tenacious discharge, a fissured eczema is the type. Great itching is always accompanying the eruption. The skin may be dry and horny. The hair is dry and falls out. Rough, hard, persistent dryness of portions of skin unaffected by eczema. Eruption oozing out a sticky exudation. Every little injury suppurates. Cracks in nipples, mouth, between toes, anus. Burning and stinging pain. Ulcers discharging a glutinous fluid, thin and sticky. Pimples and acne.

ARSENICUM : A useful remedy in all cases of skin troubles when the skin is thickened, such as in chronic eczema, psoriasis and chronic urticaria. The sensations are itching, burning and swelling, it also has papules, nettle rash and pimples. Burning sensitive ulcers with offensive discharges. It is perhaps our best general remedy for the chronic form of eczema with great burning and itching. It is almost a specific for hives from fish, which burn and for repercussed hives pustules form into scabs. Itching, burning, swellings; oedema, eruption, popular, dry, rough, scaly, worse cold and scratching. Malignant pustules. Ulcers with offensive discharge. Urticaria with burning and restlessness. Icy coldness of body. Gangrenous inflammation.

SULPHUR : The great characteristic of this remedy is the aggravation from washing; this with scratching makes the parts burn intensely. The skin is rough, coarse and there is much soreness in the fold of the skin and a tendency to pustular eruptions. Dryness and heat of scalp, with intense itching, especially at night and scratching causes soreness; wetting makes it burn. Eczema erthematosum. Eruption of yellow crusts. Eruptions at the margin of the hair. Dry, scaly, unhealthy; every little injury suppurates. Itching, burning, worse scratching and washing. Excoriation especially in folds. Feeling of a band around bones. Skin affections after local medication. Puritis especially from warmth, in evening, often occur in springtime, in damp weather.

PETROLEUM : Skin dry, constricted very sensitive, rough and cracked. Slightest scratch makes skin suppurate. Psoriasis of hands. Thick greenish crusts, burning and itching, redness, raw, cracks bleed easily. Rhagades worse in winter. Itching at night. Chilblains, moist, itch and burn. It is suited to dark skin persons who suffer from catarrhal conditions of the mucous membrane, gastric acidity and cutaneous eruptions. Ailments from riding in a carriage, cars or ships. Long lasting complaints follow mental states.

HEPAR SULPHUR : Moist eruption in folds of skin and itching in the bends of joints; the skin is extremely sensitive and suppurates easily, and pimples form around ulcers. Humid eczema of the scalp, sore and sensitive to touch. Eczema of the scrotum and genital organs boils. It is especially useful after the abuse of slaves or intents containing zinc and mercury. Suppurative glands are very sensitive. Papules prone to suppurate and extend. Acne in youth. Suppurate with prickly pain. Easily bleed. Angio-neurotic oedema. Unhealthy skin, every little injury suppurates. Chapped skin, with deep cracks on hands and feet. Ulcers with bloody suppuration. Smelling like old cheese. Ulcers very sensitive to contact, burning, stinging, and easily bleeding. Sweats day and night without relief. " Cold sores" very sensitive. Cannot bear to be uncovered; wants to be wrapped up warmly. Sticking or pricking in afflicted parts. Putrid ulcers, surrounded by little pimples. Great sensitiveness to slightest touch. Chronic and recurring urticaria. Small pox, herpes circinatus. Constant offensive exhalation from the body.

SILICIA : Felons, abscesses, boils, and old fistulous ulcers. Delicate, pale, waxy. Cracks at end of fingers. Painless swelling of glands. Rose coloured blotches. Scars suddenly become painful. Pus offensive. Promotes expulsion of foreign bodies from tissues. Every long lasting suppuration and fistulous tracts. Dry fingertips. Eruptions itch only in daytime and evening. Crippled nails. Indurated tumors. Abscesses of joints. After impure vaccination. Bursa. Lepra. Nodes and coppery spots. Keloid growths.

❑❑❑

CHAPTER 42

Rachitis

It is a constitutional disease of infancy and childhood, characterized by impairment of the general health, and arrested growth, abnormal proliferation of the developing bone.

Heredity is a frequent predisposing cause. Poor nutrition, poor housing facilities, want of cleanliness, want of sun light are both predisposing and exciting causes. Age plays a great part. Climate also has its influence, more prevalent in moist than in dry climates. Diathesis influences are second only to heredity.

Hyperemia of all the structures of the bone, periosteum, osseous tissue, cartilage and marrow, is the first step in the development of the rachitic lesion. As a result, we have proliferation of cartilage cells, retarded and irregular development of bone, softening of matrix, undue vascularity of the cancellous tissues, and weakness and deformity of the bones in various parts of the body. The weight of the bones is lessened. The vascularity of the bones is increased. In some cases the blue discoloration is due to the increased vascularity may be seen even through the thick scalp. Outside of the bones they may find blurring of striation of muscles, excessive fat in connective tissue between the muscle fibre and rare cases of fatty degeneration of the muscle fibres themselves. The liver is occasionally enlarged the spleen more rarely so.

The symptoms are seldom detected prior to the fourth month of life; increase in frequency to the end of the second year; decrease to the end of the sixth year and are seldom observed after that age. We should bear in mind, however, that the effects of the disease are seen for years afterwards, sometimes to the end of life. It is difficult to differentiate the symptoms of the active stage of the disease from those of the effects of the disease.

The family history may show syphilis, tuberculosis or some other diathesis. The condition of the mother before and during gestation may be that of over work, prolonged lactation; improper diet, or want of exercise etc. The general surroundings have been poor.

The symptoms first presented by the patient are generally referable to the digestive organs, viz, in the unnatural appetite, the abnormal stools, the enlarged abdomen, etc., followed by loss of weight. Then the patient becomes dull, listless, easily tired, inactive, emaciated or flabby. Next may be an unhealthy skin, giving us profuse offensive perspiration etc. The later symptoms, effects, the results of the disease usually make their first appearance in the thorax. They are nodules easily palpated and readily seen in the ribs with the cartilages and are due to proliferation of cartilage cells. These are not only the first, but also the most prominent results of the disease.

Important homoeopathic medicines available to cure or to prevent the rachitis in children is given below:

Homoeopathic Medicines

CALCAREA CARB is the best homoeopathic medicine. An infant of 18 months, unable to walk. There is a marked kyphosis, especially in the upper lumber region. He was pale and fretful; perhaps rather fat; but flabby. The head is usually large, with a tendency to squareness; the anterior fontanels are much more widely open than it should be at this age. The chest is ill shaped, the sternum a little more prominent and there is some constriction below the level of the nipples. The lower ribs somewhat everted above the big abdomen, in which the liver can easily be felt, and the spleen is also just palpable. The muscles feel flabby and soft just above the ankle and the wrist; the bones seem thickened. There is nothing better than Calcarea Carb 30.

CALCAREA PHOS : The hydrogenoid head i.e., brains large and heavy but the bones are thin and insufficient in quantity. A great remedy for non-union of fractured bones when due to impaired nutrition. This applies to the bones of the skull and neck. The result is: open fontanels and inability to hold up the head. The Calcarea Carb child has an abundance of bony material but the quality is poor and the amount unequally distributed. The Calcarea Carb child is dull mentally and slow in developing, but as the rule Calcarea phos child is bright, often precocious. The Calcarea Carb child is fat & flabby, but the Calcarea Phos is deficient in muscular tissue. Use Calcarea Phos 200.

CALCAREA IOD : This remedy is also good for malnutrition, when the fault lies in the glandular system. The tubercular diathesis is usually present.

The child is dark; the skin dry and unhealthy. The child is ravenously hungry but emaciation is rapid in spite of the large amount of food he takes. The mesenteric glands are always large, making the abdomen prominent. The stools are loose and offensive. Give Calcarea Iod, 200.

CHINCHONA : This homoeopathic medicine is a tonic to improve digestion and assimilation. When the patient has symptoms of painless, undigested, frothy, yellow stools. This condition follows some acute disease of the alimentary canal during which stools have been frequent and profuse, often accompanied by vomiting. The child is hungry but the food taken is not digested. This remedy will work of 30,200 potency.

SILICA : The silica child has a large head like Calcarea Phos; is emaciated like Calcarea Iod, and has a moist skin like Calcarea Carb; the stools contain undigested food like Nux Vomica and Cinchona; the diahoreaic stools are painless but very offensive. The abdomen is swollen, hot and painful. Silica is most frequently homoeopathic remedy. Curvature of bones, rickets, there is present offensive sweat. Caries after inflammation, worse from cold. Rachitis due to imperfect assimilation and consequent defective nutrition. Diseases of bones, caries and necrosis. Scrofulous, rachitic children, with large head, open fontanels and sutures, distended abdomen, slow in walking.

FLOURIC ACID : Dental fistula; caries of the bone, especially of the long bones, with thin excoriating discharge relieved by cold applications, caries of temporal bones and mastoid processes. The pains are burning and intermittent, and the discharge is thin and acrid. Caries from syphilis or mercury. Fluoric acid patient is better from cold. Early decay of teeth. Complaints of old age, or the prematurely aged, with weak distended blood vessels.

SULPHUR : Rickets, defective assimilation, great appetite, but poorly nourished. Standing is the worst position for sulphur patients, it is always uncomfortable. Dirty, filthy people, prone to skin affections. Drawing and tearing in arms and hands. Cannot walk erect; stoop shouldered.

❏❏❏

CHAPTER 43

Rheumatism

It is an inflammatory condition that mainly affects the children and young people in their teens. It is considered to be an allergic condition that mainly attacks the connective tissues of the body, causing joint pains and St. Vitus' dance due to central nervous irritation and skin lesions. The most serious damage that this disease brings is the damage to the valves does the heart. Certain streptococcus germs present in the throat are sometimes responsible.

The predisposing causes are:

1. An infective lesion, especially tonsillitis.
2. Endemic and epidemic influences.
3. Hereditary influences.
4. Climate. It occurs mostly in cities of the temperate latitudes.
5. Age 15 to 35; sex, more frequently in men than in women, and worse in February, March and April.
6. Overcrowding, malnutrition, and dampness often play some part.
7. Small outbreaks of rheumatic fever may occur in army barracks.

It usually strikes first in childhood, around eight years of age. The child comes down with a sore throat or cold, followed by an attack of tonsillitis or perhaps scarlet fever. While the patient is recovering, his one or two larger joints become red, swollen, and tender to the touch. There is also soreness in the muscles and tendons, as well as lack of appetite and a feeling of weakness. Tender nodules may appear on the skin, particularly over the joints, such as the elbows. Bleeding from the nose is common in rheumatic fever.

Pains in the chest mean that the inflammation has reached the pericardium and the heart muscle. The child may develop pneumonia, pleurisy and even abdominal pain resembling acute appendicitis. The patient may become fidgety resembling St. Vitus dance. This is more common in girls but also occur in boys. Hand movements may be rapid, jerky, and irregular and the patient has a tendency to drop things from hands. There may be muscle weakness and even some difficulty in chewing and swallowing, particularly in young girls.

In some children the disease may be of a low grade. He is easily fatigued and may not gain weight, as he should. The pulse rate may be rapid and low-grade fever may be present continuing for long periods of time. The child may complain of growing pains. This means an aching pain in the muscles and joints, and in the heart.

Many cases of the disease have no specific lesions. In few cases the synovial membrane of the affected joints are swollen and have some fibrin upon three surfaces. The serous effusion about the joint has been found sterile with few exceptions, but contains fibrin and in most cases leukocytes. The sheets of the tendons may become inflamed, the cartilages eroded and occasionally pus may be found in the exudates. Serious complications such as pericarditis, endocarditis and myocarditis may be present

General symptoms such as malaise, angina, temperature, laryngitis etc are present. Swelling of the synovial membrane of the various joints, which are tender, red and sore are present. Pain is the most important symptoms, which may be migrating, from one joint to the other from one side of the body to the other.

Cardiac complications usually come suddenly and without warning. The increase of temperature, the palpitation, the dsypnoea, the soreness and pain may be slight. Endocarditis is present in 27 to 35 percent of cases and it comes during the first ten or twelve days of the disease. The disease weakens the muscular walls and dilates the ventricles, especially the left.

A profuse, sour smelling perspiration is also an important symptom. Erythema nodosum, urticaria haemorrhagica and ecchymoses may also occur. Subcutaneous nodules, which are small, painless, firm movable, usually attached to the fascia are also present. They usually appear about the fingers, wrists, patella, ankle and elbow. They are composed of round and spindle shaped cells. They change their place from one joint to the other.

Restlessness, insomnia, delirium, melancholia, convulsions, meningitis and coma may be present. Chorea both accompanies and follows the disease, especially in children.

The urine is scanty and dark red. Urates are deposited after the urine stands for a short time. The chlorides are decreased, sometimes absent.

Homoeopathic Medicines

BRYONIA: It is the most frequently indicated and most useful remedy for acute rheumatic arthritis. It has an elective affinity for the serous membrane and muscles. Sour sweat is the characteristic symptom of Bryonia. The swelling, redness and pain are the leading indications. The pulse is rapid, face is hot and flushed, there is intense thirst, there is dirty white coating on the tongue, urine is dark and scanty, loss of appetite, the hard, dry, dark stools. The muscles are sore and swollen and the joints are violently inflamed, red and swollen, shiny and very hot. The pains are sharp, stitching, or cutting in character. It prefers the right side, the evening and the open air. Bryonia affects especially the constitution of a robust, firm fiber and dark complexion, with tendency to leanness and irritability.

RHUS TOX : Rheumatic pains spread over a large surface at nape of neck, loins and extremities; better by motion. Soreness of condyles of bones. Limbs stiff, paralyzed. Numbness and formication after over work and exposure. Paralysis, trembling after exertion. Tenderness about knee joint. Loss of power in forearm and fingers. The cold fresh air is not tolerated it makes the joints painful. Ailments from strains, over lifting, getting wet while perspiring. Aggravation from rest and over exertion and amelioration from change of position and heat are the ranking modalities of Rhustox.

LEDUM : We have the symptoms that the ball of the great toe is swollen, sore and painful on stepping; drawing pains worse from warmth, pressure and from motion. It has also gouty nodosities in the joints. All the pains of the Ledum travel upwards. Throbbing in right shoulder. Cracking in joints worse from warmth of bed. Ankles swollen. Easy spraining of ankle. Soles painful, can hardly step on them. There is a general lack of animal heat, and yet heat of bed is in tolerable. Ledum mainly acts on the small joints. It is an excellent remedy in erythema nodosum, which is of the rheumatic origin. Wine aggravates all the symptoms of this remedy. The effusion into the joints is scanty and it soon hardens to form the nodosities.

COLCHICUM : The typical case calling for Colchicum is where the swelling is red or pale, with extreme tenderness to touch, a tendency to shift about from joint to joint, and pains which are worse on the slightest motion. If the general symptoms of great prostration of the muscular system and abdominal bloating is present Colchicum is the remedy. It is also characterized by the gastric symptoms and cardiac complications. It is more indicated when the smaller joints, fingers, toes, wrists and ankles are affected; the pains are very violent, patient cannot bear to have the parts touched or to have anyone come near him, the Colchicum patient is apt to be exceedingly irritable and the gout is not apt to decrease this irritability. There is always great prostration, internal coldness and tendency to collapse. Limbs lame, weak, tingling, tearing in limbs during warm weather, stinging during cold. Oedematous swelling and coldness of legs and feet.

□□□

CHAPTER 44

Sepsis

It is caused by the entry of the bacteria in to the blood.

The pathogenetic bacteria or their products usually enter the blood through some break in the skin or mucous membrane. Although sepsis may be more easily traced to infection through tears in the parturient canal and other wounds, yet many cases have their origin in the respiratory organs, digestive tract including the teeth and other organs or tissues. Suppuration in any part of the body like otitis, dental or rectal fistula may give rise to sepsis. Gonorrhea or the infections may be directly the cause of sepsis or indirectly by leaving channels for the invading organisms. The most frequent organisms are the staphylococci, although ten or twelve others have been found. Sepsis affects both sexes and all ages.

In the pyemic cases, the abscesses, emboli, thrombi, degeneration of the surrounding tissues, etc., were found most frequently in the lungs then kidneys, spleen and liver. Changes found: blood dark and disintegrated; spleen large and soft; fatty degeneration of the heart; kidney large, pale with prechynmatous changes; liver large with fatty degeneration.

The order of the appearance and severity of symptoms varies greatly not only in the different forms of sepsis but also in individuals suffering from the same form. This makes the treatment of the patient rather than the treatment of the disease, imperative. A patient suffering from a certain cocci infection with a different cocci serum or a patient calling for Arsenicum or Baptisia. A septic focus before the pus gets into the blood stream. Certain bacteria may start a conflagration within a few hours after invading the blood current.

Some symptoms are generally present like: chillness or chill followed by a sudden rise in temperature, headache, nausea, malaise etc., may have been present for days or even weeks before the rise in temperature appears. In some cases temperature may remain the high without intermission. In others, temperature may be remittent or intermittent, or the temperature may be atypical typhoid one. In some cases the skin is dry, in others skin is bathed with profuse sweat, or dryness or moisture may alternate. The pulse however is more reliable. It gradually becomes rapid and weak. The patient may be apathetic or very restless; the patient may be violently delirious or the delirium may be of a low type. The joints are sometimes painful. The spleen is often enlarged and tender, also the liver. Emaciation is rapid. The sunken eyes, drawn face and the petechial or purpuric eruption of the skin in other parts of the body are often present. Disturbances of the alimentary tract, i.e., nausea, vomiting, constipation, etc. are frequent symptoms.

Some of the important homoeopathic medicines are given below:

Homoeopathic Medicines

LACHESIS : This remedy does its best work in localized pyaemia, traumatic gangrene and carbuncles. Indications are blue skin, sensitive parts, great prostration and scanty discharges. It has the prostration of arsenic but lacks its restlessness. In low conditions of abscess when the pus is thin, dark, ichorus and offensive in character. It is the remedy for abscess where poisonous matter has been introduced into the system, causing the trouble. The great debility, the production of watery, ichorus pus the threatening of gangrene and the intolerable itching, burning pains are the characteristic of this remedy.

RHUS TOXCODENDRON: Produces a perfect picture of septicemia, with redness and soreness at the point of infection. Chillness, dry tongue, diarrohea and restlessness. It is a very useful remedy in acute suppuration: especially it has been found useful in suppurative conditions about the eye. It has been proved curative in abscesses about the parotid and axillary glands: the pus is bloody and serous, the pain is intense, and the swelling is dark red. Glands swollen. Burning eczematous eruptions with tendency to scale formation.

CARBOLIC ACID: This internally is a neglected remedy in septicemia. Prostration exhaustion to the point of collapse is indications. The patient falls asleep from weariness and wakens unrefreshed. Pains are terrible, come and go suddenly. Physical exertion brings on abscess somewhere. Putrid discharges. Scarlet fever, with marked tendency to destruction of tissue internally, and fetid odor. Itching vesicles, with burning pain. Burns tend to ulcerate.

BELLADONNA : It is the remedy most often indicated for the initiatory symptoms of sepsis and abscess. The parts swell rapidly, becomes bright red, there is intense throbbing, which is painful, pus develops speedily, the swelling increases and redness radiates. It comes in earlier than either of these remedies and corresponds more closely to the active, asthenic variety of abscess before pus is matured. In abscesses about the alveolar processes, gumboils, belladonna is the first remedy. In acute glandular abscesses Belladonna is often indicated and is the first remedy. Alternate redness and paleness of the skin. Indurations after inflammations. Skin is dry and hot: swollen, sensitive, burns, scarlet, smooth. Suppurative wounds.

HEPAR SULPHUR : It is the great homoeopathic medicine for suppurations where the pus is not decomposed. Excessive sensitiveness of the parts is a leading indication. Chilly sensations, throbbing in the parts, or sharp sticking pains, which are worse at night and from cold. Hepar if given in the higher potencies will often abort the suppurative process. Hepar cures such abscesses such as felon and whitlow very well. Suppurating glands are very sensitive. Papules prone to suppurate and extend. Suppurate with prickly pain. Unhealthy skin, every little injury suppurates. Ulcers, with bloody suppuration, smelling like old cheese. Ulcers very sensitive to contact, burning, stinging, and easily bleeding. Sweats day and night without relief. Cannot bear to be uncovered; wants to be wrapped up warmly. Putrid ulcers, surrounded by little pimples.

SILICEA : It is the remedy where the suppuration continues and the wound refuses to heal, no matter where the suppurative process is located, the pus is apt to be thin, watery and the process is a sluggish and indolent one. In Silicea the suppurative process takes on a healthy patient, the pus becomes benign, granulations appear. Warmth is very grateful to the Silicea patient. Abscesses having much cellular infiltration also call for this remedy. It is also a remedy for fistulous ulcers. In rectal fistula it is very often the remedy, great nervous tension is present. The discharge from the abscess is very fetid. Scrofulous and tubercular abscesses especially call for this remedy. Painless swelling of glands. Pus offensive. Promotes expulsion of foreign bodies from tissues. Every little injury suppurates. Long lasting suppuration and fistulous tracts. Eruptions itch only in daytime and evening. Abscess of joints.

MERCURIUS : It is a very good remedy for abscess. It favors the formation of pus especially in lower potencies, indicated in glandular abscesses; the pus is greenish, thin and fluid. There is intense, shining redness with throbbing and stinging pains. It is one of the best medicines for abscesses at the root of the teeth and is often indicated in toothache due to abscess. It will often abort suppurative process when used in higher potencies, as in tonsillitis, where it is the most suitable remedy. It is a remarkable remedy in pyorrhea and will make extraction of teeth unnecessary. Excessive odorous viscid perspiration; worse night. General tendency to free perspiration, but patient is not relieved thereby. Vesicular and pustular eruptions. Ulcers irregular in shape, edges undefined. Pimples around the main eruption. Itching, worse from warmth of bed.

❑❑❑

CHAPTER 45

Sexual Impotency

MALE STERLITY, or failure to fertilize female egg cells, may be due to several causes. In some cases the trouble is due to an emotional factor, such as a mental block. It may be caused by an absence or atrophy of the testes, or perhaps by some obstruction in the male genital organs. Infections involving the 'genital organs may result in the production of unhealthy or even dead sperm cells. In such cases special tests may locate the seat of the trouble, which may be treated surgically.

FEMALE STERLITY, or failure to have children may arise from several different causes. Sometimes the trouble is due to the husband.

The ovum remains viable and capable of being fertilized after it is expelled from the ovary probably no longer than 24 hours. Therefore, sperm must be available soon after ovulation if fertilization is to take place. On the other hand, a few sperm can remain fertile in the female reproductive tract for up to 72 hours, although most of them for not more than 24 hours. Therefore fertilization to take place, intercourse usually must occur sometime between 1 to 2 days before ovulation and up to 1 day after ovulation

In a woman, sterility may be due to some congenital malformation that has existed from birth, such as an absence of the tubes, ovary or uterus. Such conditions are rare. Pelvic infections, involving the vagina or cervix, are a more common cause of sterility. Inflammation of the tubes may prevent the sperm from reaching the ovum.

Other conditions such as endometriosis and adhesions involving the genital organs may also interfere with pregnancy. Endometriosis causes fibrosis throughout the pelvis and this fibrosis sometimes so covers the ovaries that an ovum cannot be released into the abdominal cavity. Endometriosis also occludes the fallopian tubes either at the fimbriated ends or else where along their extent. Lack of a normal menstrual cycle may also be a factor. In some cases, the real cause of sterility arises from emotional factors. Many women who have waited for years for a family of their own have adopted a baby and then found themselves pregnant a few months later. The very presence of a baby in home apparently releases powerful maternal forces within the woman, thus solving her problem. Still another cause of infertility is secretion of abnormal mucus by the uterine cervix. Abnormalities of the cervix itself, such as low-grade infection or inflammation, or abnormal hormonal stimulation of the cervix can lead to a viscous mucus plug that will prevent fertilization.

It has been known that the administration of either estrogen or progesterone, if given in appropriate quantity during the first half of the monthly female cycle, can inhibit ovulation. The reason for this is that appropriate administration of either of these hormones can prevent the preovulatory surge of LH secretion by the pituitary gland, which is essential in causing ovulation.

The most common cause of female sterility is failure to ovulate. This can result from hypo secretion of gonadotropic hormones; in such cases the intensity of the hormonal stimuli is not sufficient to cause ovulation. For example, thick capsules occasionally exist on the outside of the ovaries that make ovulation difficult.

Treatment in homoeopathy is available for both male and female infertility. Some of the medicines with their symptoms are given below:

Homoeopathic Medicines

PHOSPHORIC ACID : The remedy corresponds to the chronic effects of loss of seminal fluids. The whole system is weakened; the legs are weak, and there is burning in the spine worse at night, the genitals are relaxed, the scrotum and testicles are flabby, the penis has no power of erection, or the erections are imperfect and the semen escapes too soon during coitus. Formication or a sensation of crawling on the scrotum is also sometimes present. Impotency when the sensibility of the part is excessive, and the semen is discharged shortly after or even before erection. There is a sudden relaxation of the penis during coitus due to exhaustion rather than to spasmodic action. There is dragging in the testicals.

STAPHISGARIA : It is the remedy for the bad effects of masturbation where there is great emaciation with dark rings under the eyes, sallow face, peevishness and shyness. The patient is hypochondriac and permits the mind to dwell too long on sexual subjects; the boy becomes apathetic and gloomy, he has sunken face and he becomes uneasy about the state of his health. There may be irritability of the prostatic portion of the urethra. In the female, Staphysgaria is the remedy when the organs are in a state of irritability. It is the remedy in anxious and imaginary persons who are uneasy about the state of the health. In females parts are very sensitive, worse sitting down.

NUX VOMICA : It is indicated for the bad effects of early masturbation. It should be given when the patient suffers from headache; frequent involuntary emissions at night, especially toward morning, and the digestive organs are weak. There is an irritable condition from sexual excesses, erections taking place. Nux patients are easily chilled, avoid open air. Nux is preeminently the remedy for many of the conditions incident to modern life. The typical nux patient is rather thin, quick, active, nervous and irritable.

SEPIA : Sepia is remedy acting especially on the female organs and is a most valuable one. There is weakness and want of tone in the whole body, the yellow complexion, the yellow saddle over the nose, the sunken dark-ringed eyes, the relief from violent motion and amelioration in the middle of the day. The menses are late and scanty. The leucorrhoea of Sepia is yellow green in color and somewhat offensive. It may be milky; it is worse before the menses and is accompanied by bearing down. The uterus is enlarged and the cervix is indurated. Bearing down pains is the most important characteristic of the remedy and sitting relieves this sensation with the limbs crossed. There is also a severe lumbo sacral backache. It has great dryness of the vulva and vagina, painful to touch. It is a useful remedy for ovaritis with dull, heavy pains.

LILIUM TIGRINUM: The leucorrhoea is watery, yellow or yellowish brown and excoriating. There is much nervousness and aimless hurrying; the mind and body are weak and patients lack self-confidence in themselves; restless, weakness is characteristic. There are ovarian pains more severe on the left side, shooting down anterior and inner aspect of thigh.

PLATINUM: The pride, he haughtiness, the self-esteem and the belittling of everyone are found in the remedy. The menses are profuse and clotted and occurs too early, with much sensitiveness about the genitals. There is constant irritation about the sexual organs, both internally and externally. It is also a remedy for indurations and prolapse of the uterus, where there is pressure in the groin and back with sensitiveness of the parts to the touch. It is one of the important remedies for painful coitus. It is also useful in ovaritis with burning pains and numbness of the limbs.

❏❏❏

CHAPTER 46

Sinusitis

Sinusitis or accessory sinus suppuration is bacterial inflammation of the nasal and contiguous sinuses following acute rhinitis especially streptococci. Sometimes the infection travels from the second bicuspid and first two molar teeth whose roots are near to the antral floor. Sinusitis is an important etiological factor in the causation of many diseases of the lower respiratory tract.

Inflammation of the paranasal sinuses often follows the common cold, influenza, and other general infections. Germs that would normally be eliminated from the body may sometimes find their way into these little sinuses or chambers on each side of the nasal passages. Trouble may be due to inadequate drainage resulting from a deviated septum, or perhaps to the presence of polyps. Any chronic infection within the nose may lead to sinuses.

Acute Sinusitis is characterized by moderate degree of fever and local pain. The latter depends on the site affected: if frontal sinus, forehead; antrum, on one cheek: sphenoidal sinus, deep-seated headache. Headache is more marked in the afternoon.

Exposure to marked changes in temperature and humidity may also result in generalized inflammation within the nose, and this may extend into the sinuses. Dental abscesses may find their way into the maxillary sinuses, which are located on each side of the nose just above the jaw.

There is a purulent nasal discharge and in some cases, epistaxis. A progressive ill health continues. The patient usually complains of headache, postnatal discharge, pain and perhaps a low-grade fever, lack of appetite, loss of smell and even toothache. The trouble usually begins in one sinus and unless checked it may soon spread to other areas. Most cases clear up rapidly under good treatment, but some go on to the chronic stage. Sinus headaches are usually felt in the forehead and behind the eyes, or in the face just below the eyes. Many patients think they are having frequent colds, when in reality the trouble is due to recurrent sinus infection.

The infection may extent to the eyes, ears, throat and tracheo- bronchial tree: occasionally intracranial complications as meningitis, cavernous sinus thrombosis and brain abscess may appear.

In severe cases of sinusitis, the inside of the nose appears boggy and red and may be covered with a thin layer of pus. X-rays of the sinuses may show the presence of fluid or even polyps growing inside the involved sinus. The inflammation may also cause a severe infection of the middle ear, as well as bronchopneumonia, asthmatic attacks and even an abscess of the brain in rare cases.

Chronic sinus infection may not cause any definite symptoms except during exacerbations. This is frequently associated with many chronic respiratory infections.

Homoeopathic Medicines

HEPAR SULPH : Soreness of the nostrils, with catarrhal troubles. Sneezes every time he goes into a cold, dry wind with running from nose later, thick, offensive discharge. Stopped up nose every time he goes out into cold air. Smell like old cheese. Yellowish complexion of the face. Neuralgia of right side of face, extending in streak into temple. When swallowing sensation of a plug and of a splinter in throat. Stitches in throat extending to the ear when swallowing. Hawking up of mucus. Great sensitiveness to all impressions. Sweating patient pulling blanket around him. Infected sinus with pus forming. The tendency to suppuration is most marked. Chilliness, hypersensitiveness, splinter like pains, craving for sour and strong things are very characteristic.

KALI BICHROMICUM : Pressure and pain at root of nose, and sticking pain in nose. Septum ulcerated; round ulcer. Fetid smell. Discharge thick, ropy, greenish yellow. Tough elastic plugs from nose; leave a raw surface. Inflammation extends to frontal sinuses, with distress and fullness at root of nose. Dropping from posterior nares. Loss of smell. Much hawking. Inability to breathe through nose. Dryness. Coryza with obstruction of nose. Violent sneezing. Profuse, watery nasal discharge. Chronic inflammation of frontal sinus with stopped up sensation. Blotchy red appearance. Bones sensitive, especially beneath orbits. Discharge from mouth and throat, tough and stringy.

HYDRASTIS : Thick, tenacious secretion from posterior nares to throat. Watery, excoriating discharge. Ozaena with ulceration of septum. Tends to blow nose all the time. Follicular pharyngitis. Raw, smarting excoriating sensation. Hawking of yellow, tenacious mucus. Child is aroused suddenly from sleep by this tenacious post-nasal dropping. Chest raw, sore, burning. Dry, hash cough. Frequent faintly spells, with cold sweat all over. Feels suffocating when lying on left side. Pain from chest to left shoulder.

PHOSPHORUS : Fan like motion of nostrils. Bleeding; epistaxis instead of menses. Oversensitive to smell. Periostitis of nasal bones. Foul imaginary odours. Chronic catarrh with small haemorrhages; handkerchief is always bloody. Polyp, bleeding easily. Sickly, pale complexion of the face, blue rings under the eyes. Dryness in pharynx and fauces. Thirst for very cold water. It is suited to tall, slender persons, narrow chested, with thin transparent skin, weakened by loss of animal fluids, with great nervous debility and emaciation. Phosphorus irritates, inflames and degenerates mucous membranes, irritates and inflames serous membranes.

NUX VOMICA : There is rough, scraped feeling in the throat. Tickling in throat after waking in morning. Sensation of roughness, tightness and tension. Pharynx constricted. Uvula swollen. Stitches into ear. Nose is stuffed at night. Stuffy colds, snuffles after exposure to dry, cold atmosphere; worse in warm room. Odors tend to produce fainting. Coryza is fluent in daytime, stuffed at night and outdoors. Bleeding in morning. Acrid discharge, but with stuffed up feeling. First half of tongue clean; posterior covered with deep fur, white yellow, cracked edges.

SABADILLA : The important characteristic symptoms of this remedy are sore throat worse on left side. Tough phlegm. Sensation of a skin hanging loosely must swallow it. Warm food and drink relieve. Empty swallowing most painful. Dry fauces and throat. Sensation of a lump in throat with constant necessity to swallow. Chronic sore throat; worse from cold air. Spasmodic sneezing, with running nose. Coryza with severe frontal pains and redness of eyes and lacrymation. Copious watery nasal discharge. Action on mucous membranes of the nose and the lachrymal glands producing coryza and symptoms like hay fever are the characteristic symptoms of this remedy.

SILICEA : There is pricking as of a pin in tonsil. Cold settles in throat. Parotids glands swollen. Stinging pain on swallowing. Hard, cold swelling of cervical glands. Sensation of hair on tongue. Facial neuralgia, throbbing, tearing, face red, worse cold damp. Itching at point of nose. Dry, hard crusts form, bleeding when loosened. Nasal bones sensitive. Sneezing in morning. Nose obstructed and loss of smell. Perforation of septum.

CHAPTER 47

Sore Throat

The pharynx, or back of the throat, frequently becomes inflamed when a person has a cold or an attack of influenza. This inflammation may also involve the tonsils and adenoids if these have not already been removed.

This is due to many causes:

i) Inflammation of the fauces, soft palate and uvula.

a) Catarrh along with acute tonsillitis

b) Gummatous ulcerations

c) Tuberculosis

d) Carcinoma

ii) Tonsils

a) Acute inflammation: diphtheritic, streptococcal, syphilitic, pneumococcal, or a complication of influenza, rheumatic fever, measles and other eruptive fevers.

b) Chronic hypertrophied tonsils-adenoids, syphilitic or tuberculous affections or new growth.

ii) Pharynx

a) Acute catarrh

b) Septic or

c) Chronic granular pharyngitis

d) Post pharyngeal abscess

e) Inflammation as a complication of eruptive fevers and]

f) Carcinoma

iii) Larynx

a) Acute catarrhal or inhalation of irritants

The symptoms are those of a simple irritation or inflammation to those of granulation and ulceration. The subjective symptoms are dryness, fullness, chilliness, frequent desire to swallow and occasionally a sense of suffocation; sharp, sticking, splinter like pain in the ulcerative form. The objective symptoms are a red, dry surface at first and later granules, follicles, ulcers; muco and mucopurulent secretions; hawked up after coughing and some fever. The skin is usually dry and the patient is constipated. Lymph glands along the sides of the neck may become swollen and tender. Swallowing may be difficult, especially during the acute stage. If the irritation has extended up into the nasal passages, there will also be a thick postnasal discharge.

Homoeopathic Medicines

BELLADONNA. : This remedy corresponds to many sore throats and is very often prescribed. It is indicated by great dryness and brightness of the throat; it has glazed appearance, the fauces are inflamed, the tonsils are swollen and enlarged, worse on right side; constant desire to swallow. There is constricted sensation in the throat, worse from swallowing when liquids and even food are ejected through the nose. There is great soreness from the swelling and hyperasthesia of the fauces. Sore throats and catarrhal origin rapid in progress and having dryness are important indications for Belladonna. The patient is drowsy, the patient does not sleep. Cough is spasmodic and the child cries after each paroxysm. Larynx feel sore. Cheyne-stokes breathing. Cough with pain in left hip. Barking cough, whooping cough, with pain in stomach before attack, with expectoration of blood. Larynx very painful. Stitches in chest when coughing. Respiration oppressed, quick, unequal.

MERCURIUS : It has great dryness and soreness of the throat, the patient is obliged to swallow constantly and there is much soreness and swelling of the glands externally. The throat is raw and burning and also red and swollen. It is useful in sub acute or torpid anginas and in affections of the throat appearing on every change of weather. An offensive breathe from the mouth is a guiding symptom. Bluish red swelling. Constant desire to swallow. Putrid sore throat; worse right side. Ulcers and inflammation appearing at every change of weather. Stitches into ear on swallowing. Quinsy with difficult swallowing after pus has formed. Sore, raw, smarting, burning throat. Complete loss of voice. Burning in throat, as from hot vapor ascending.

PHYTOLACCA : It is indicated where the throat is dark red in colour and the tonsils are also red in colour, the parts feel sore, and the pain on swallowing is at the root of the tongue accompanied by a general aching in the back and limbs. It suits chronic follicular pharyngitis where there is present a constant desire to clear the throat of phlegm or a sensation of a hot ball in the throat worse from hot fluids. The right side is more frequently affected. Much pain at the root of the tongue; soft palate and tonsils swollen. Sensation of a lump in throat. Throat feels rough, narrow, and hot. Shooting pain into ears on swallowing. Pseudomembranous exudations, grayish white, thick, tenacious yellowish mucus, difficult to dislodge. Tension and pressure in parotid gland. Uvula large, dropsical. Quinsy; tonsils and fauces swollen with burning pain cannot swallow even water.

LACHESIS : Sensation of a lump in the throat, which seems to go down when swallowing, but remains again; constriction of throat and difficult breathing, worse arousing from sleep or after sleep. Empty swallowing is painful and fluids escape from the nose; the throat is sensitive externally, and though the throat is bluish red the discomfort is much greater than the appearance of the parts would indicate. It is also indicated for irritable and nervous sore throats. Sore, worse left side, swallowing liquids. Septic parotiditis. Dry, intensely swollen, externally and internally. Chronic sore throat with much hawking; mucus sticks and cannot be forced up or down. Very painful; worse slightest pressure, touch is even more painful. Purple livid colour of the throat. Feeling as if something was swollen which must be swallowed; worse swallowing saliva or liquids. Pain into ear. Collar and neck band must be very loose.

KALI BICHROMICUM : Sore throat, with swelling of the tonsils and ulcers which exude a purulent discharge; there are diseased follicles which exude a caseaous matter; the coating of the tongue is yellow at the base; there is accumulation of the sticky tenacious mucus in the pharynx and pain in the Eustachian tubes. There is a sensation of dryness, of burning and of rawness, or a scraping feeling as if something were sticking in the throat. Fauces red and inflamed. Parotid glands swollen. Uvula relaxed, oedematous bladder like. Pseudomembranous deposits on tonsils and soft palate. Burning extending to stomach. Discharge from mouth and throat tough and stringy.

HEPAR SULPH : Sharp splinter like pains in the throat indicate this remedy, or a sensation as if there were a lump in the throat. Suppurative throat troubles, tonsillitis and retropharangeal abscess. The sensation of a fish bone in the throat. Nitric acid has a sensation of splinter like in the throat. Quinsy with impending suppuration. Stitches in throat extending to ear when swallowing. Hawking up of mucus.

CHAPTER 48

Sunstroke

Sunstroke results from direct heat rays of the sun. The victim may be mentally confused and complain of a bad headache. He may become delirious. His blood pressure may fall to a low level and the pulse become rapid and weak. An abnormal condition due to exposure to excessive heat.

The predisposing cause is anything, which lowers normal resistance; the chief of which are worry, excitement, mental or physical fatigue, alcoholic excesses, and lack of nourishment etc.

The exciting causes are prolonged exposure under the direct rays of the sun, unusual exertion in a hot, moist, sultry, breezeless atmosphere. The occupations, which furnish most of the cases, are breakers, boiler tenders, soldiers on the march, masons etc.

Different stages, or forms or different degrees of severity of the same condition have produced different results and been given different names, viz., heatstroke, sunstroke, heat exhaustion, insulation, thermic fever, heat prostration.

Our post-mortems show early and marked rigor mortis: putrefaction changes take place; in the brain, cerebral and spinal membranes show marked venous engorgement; the blood is darker than normal and has lost its tendency to form rouleaux, the corpusles are crenated. An acute paranchymatous degeneration of the neurons of the entire neural axis similar to that of " A species of auto-intoxication "

Symptoms vary according to the stage of the disease as well as the form. In the asphyxia form, heat apoplexy, which fortunately is rare. The most pronounced cases are those of patients working in the sun who suddenly fall unconscious, may or may not have a few convulsions, and die. Others may have some prodromal symptoms or premonitions like dizziness; throbbing, splitting headache; red flushed face; dry hot skin; full rapid pulse etc. Then comes the sudden loss of consciousness, which in fatal cases is followed by coma, which becomes more & more marked till death. In some cases Cheynestokes respiration may precede death.

Most cases are sudden in their attack, some do have prodromes such as frequent attacks of dizziness; bursting, splitting headache; coloured vision, blurred vision; hot skin alternating moist and dry; flushed face; suffused eyes; pupils dilated or pin-point; weakness; restlessness; irritability.

Heat exhaustion may present all the symptoms just enumerated, and then the skin becomes cold, clammy and pale, the pulse small and rapid; the temperature may fall as low as 95, urine suppressed or scanty.

WHAT TO DO : Carry the victim to a cool place as quickly as possible. Keep him lying down. Remove his outer clothing and apply ice bags or cold cloths to the head and neck, to help cool the brain and restore the temperature to normal. If possible wrap the patient in a wet sheet and then pour cold water over him frequently until the skin resumes its normal color. Rub or massage the limbs in the direction of the heart to aid circulation.

For severe cases of sunstroke homeopathic medicines are available. Symptoms of few medicines are given below:

Homoeopathic Medicines

GLONINE : This is the most important remedy for sunstroke. The indications for the use of this medicine are pale face, fixed eyes, white tongue, full, round pulse, labored respiration, cerebral vomiting and sinking at the pit of the stomach. The temperature is high and often times there is unconsciousness. It is also suitable for the after effects of the sunstroke. Great remedy for congestive headaches, hyperaemia of the brain from excess of heat. Children get sick when sitting in an open fire. Violent convulsions, associated with cerebral congestion. Sun headache, increases and decreases with the sun. Effects of sunstroke; heat on head, as in typesetters and workers under gas and electric light. Head heavy but cannot lay it on pillow. Cannot bear any heat about head. Better from uncovering head. Throbbing headache. Vertigo on assuming upright position. Head feels enormously large, as if skull were too small for brain.

BELLADONNA : There is drowsiness, loss of consciousness, whizzing in the ears and constriction of the chest. The headache is violent, pounding, throbbing, relieved by cold applications or having the head high. The face is flushed, the pulse full and bounding. Vertigo with falling to left side or backwards. Sensitive to least contact. Much throbbing and heat. Headache from suppressed catarrhal flow. Pain worse light, noise, jar, lying down and in afternoon; better by pressure and semi erect posture. Headache worse on right side and when lying down; ill effects, colds, etc. from having hair cut. , The temperature of the skin is increased, the skin may be moist or dry, the eyeballs are prominent, pain deep in the eyeballs, the pupils dilated, the mucous membrane dry, the lids stiff, swollen and dry; occasionally the Belladonna patient will have some tremors.

NATRUM CARB : This remedy is particularly useful in the chronic effects of sunstroke and in headaches, which return in hot weather. Natrum carb will sometimes calm very excitable and nervous persons during thunderstorms. It is also a useful remedy in debility and headache from the sun. Pain in head from slightest mental exertion, worse from sun or working under gaslight. Head feels too large. Oversensitive of hearing. Vertigo from exposure to sun. Great debility caused by summer heat; exhaustion; anaemia; milky watery skin.

ACONITE : It is a useful remedy in sunstroke where the great heat seems to have a paralyzing influence on the circulation. Fullness; heavy, pulsating, hot, bursting, burning, undulating sensation. Intracranial pressure. Burning headache as if boiling water moved brain. Vertigo worse on rising and shaking head. Sensation on vertex as if hair were pulled or stood on end. Eyes red and hot, feels dry and hot as if sand in them. Very sensitive to noises; music is unbearable.

LACHESIS : The sun's heat makes the patient dizzy and faint; hot weather greatly fatigues. Pain through head on awaking. Pain at root of nose. Pressure and burning on vertex. Waves of pain; worse after moving. Sun headache. With headache, flickering, dim vision, very pale face. Vertigo, relieved by onset of a discharge. Sensation as if eyes were drawn together by cords which were tied in a knot at root of nose. Face is purple, mottled, puffed; looks swollen and bloated.

□□□

CHAPTER 49

Stress

Stress and depression can ruin your life and affect your health. Seeking support, being realistic and planning ahead can help ward off stress and depression.

For some people, the holidays bring unwelcome guests – stress and depression. And it's no wonder. In an effort to pull off a perfect Hallmark holiday, you might find yourself facing a dizzying array of demands – work, parties, shopping, baking, cleaning, caring for kids on school break or elderly parents, and scores of other chores. So much for peace and joy, right?

Holiday stress and depression are often the result of three main trigger points. Understanding these trigger points can help you plan ahead on how to accommodate them.

Here are the three issues that commonly trigger holiday stress or depression:

- *Finances* : Like your relationships, your financial situation can cause stress at any time of the year. Overspending during the holidays on gifts, travel, food and entertainment can increase stress as you try to make ends meet while ensuring that everyone on your shopping list is happy.
- *Relationships* : Relationships can cause tension, conflict or stress at any time. But tensions are often increased during the holidays. Family misunderstandings and conflict can intensify – especially if you're all together for several days. A conflict mainly arises with so increased needs and interests to accommodate. On the other hand, if you're facing the holidays without a loved one, you may find yourself especially lonely or sad.

- *Physical demands* : The strain of shopping, attending social gatherings and preparing holiday meals can also create problems. Feeling exhausted can increase your stress, creating a vicious cycle. Exercise and sleep – good antidotes for stress and fatigue – may take a back seat to chores and errands. High demands, stress, lack of exercise, and overindulgence in food and drink – these are the ingredients for holiday illness.

When stress is at its peak, it's hard to stop and regroup. Take steps to help prevent normal holiday depression from progressing into chronic depression. Try these tips:

- *Acknowledge your feelings* : If a loved one has recently died or you aren't near loved ones, realize that it's normal to feel sadness and grief. It's OK now and then to take time just to cry or express your feelings. You don't have to force yourself to be happy just because it's the holiday season.
- *Seek support* : If you feel isolated or down, seek out family members and friends, or community, religious or social services. They can offer support and companionship. Getting involved and helping others can lift your spirits and broaden your social circle. Also, enlist support for organizing holiday gatherings, as well as meal preparation and cleanup. You don't have to go it alone.
- *Be realistic* : As families change and grow, traditions often change as well. Hold on to those you can, if you want to. But understand that in some cases that may no longer be possible. Perhaps your entire extended family can't gather together at your house. Instead, find new ways to celebrate together from afar, such as sharing pictures, e-mails or videotapes.
- *Set differences aside* : Try to accept family members and friends as they are, even if they don't live up to your expectations. Set aside grievances until a more appropriate time for discussion. With stress and activity levels high, the holidays might not be conducive to making quality time for relationships. And be understanding if others get upset or distressed. Chances are, they're feeling the effects of holiday stress, too.
- *Stick to a budget* : Before you go shopping, decide how much money you can afford to spend on gifts and other items. Then be sure to stick to your budget. If you don't, you could feel anxious and tense for months afterward as you struggle to pay the bills.
- *Plan ahead* : Set aside specific days for shopping, baking, visiting friends and other activities. Plan your menus. That'll help prevent a last-minute

scramble to buy forgotten ingredients – and you'll have time to make another pie if the first one's a flop. Allow extra time for travel so that delays won't worsen your stress.

- *Learn to say no* : Believe it or not, people will understand if you can't do certain projects or activities. If you say yes only to what you really want to do, you'll avoid feeling resentful and overwhelmed. If it's really not possible to say no to something – your boss asks you to work overtime – try to remove something from your agenda to make up for the lost time.
- *Don't abandon healthy habits* : Don't let the holidays become a dietary free-for-all. Some indulgence is OK, but overindulgence may add to your stress and guilt. Have a healthy snack before holiday parties so that you don't go overboard on sweets, cheese or drinks. Continue to get plenty of sleep and schedule time for physical activity.
- *Take a breather* : While you may not have time every day for a silent night, make some time for yourself. Spending just 15 minutes alone, without distractions, may refresh you enough to handle everything you need to do. Go away to a silent place, even if it's the bathroom, for a few moments of solitude. Take a walk at night. Listen to light music. Find something that clears your mind, slows your breathing and restores your calm.
- *Rethink resolutions* : Resolutions can set you up for failure if they're unrealistic. Don't resolve to change your whole life to make up for past excess. Instead, try to return to basic, healthy lifestyle routines. Set smaller, more specific goals with a reasonable time frame. Choose resolutions that help you feel valuable and provide more than only fleeting moments of happiness.
- *Forget about perfection* : Holiday TV specials are filled with happy endings. But in real life, people don't usually resolve problems within an hour or two. Something always comes up. You may get stuck late at the office and miss your daughter's school play, you may forget to put nuts in the cake, and your mother may criticize how you and your partner are raising the kids. All in the same day. Expect and accept imperfections.
- Seek professional help if you need it. Despite your best efforts, you may find yourself feeling sad or anxious, diseased by physical complaints, unable to sleep, irritable and hopeless, and unable to face routine works. If these feelings last for several weeks, talk to your doctor or a mental health professional. You may have depression.

Remember, one key to minimizing holiday stress and depression knows that the holidays can trigger stress and depression. Accept that things aren't always going to go as planned. Then take active steps to manage stress and depression during the holidays. You may actually enjoy the holidays this year more than you thought you could.

Besides these tips there are homoeopathic medicines available which are helpful in curing the stress. These are given below:

Homoeopathic Medicines

IGNATIA : Most cases of stress at sometime or the other require this medicine. It suits to women better. The ignatia patient is sad, with a tendency to weep. She hides her grief, is changeable and silent. It is a remedy full of disappointment and jealousy and is most suitable to complaints arising from fear, grief, and shock or prolonged weeping over real or imaginary troubles. They refuse sympathy, but feel neglected by friends. The patient has a tendency to weep over her sorrows, is intolerant to noise and tends to fixed ideas. There are sharp piercing pains in the side of the head. The cause of the headache is usually grief, or some real or imaginary insult. The accompanying symptoms are: Frequent desire to urinate, the urine may be very profuse or scanty. The odor of the urine is pungent.

NUX VOMICA : This remedy is mainly indicated for businessmen of sedentary habits. They cannot bear to be opposed, are irritable and easily angered. It is suited to men of low temper where there is great inclination to mental work. The patient resists everything done for her, with no interest in anything, offensive breath. The nux patient is oversensitive, sad mostly due to digestive and hepatic troubles. The typical nux patient is rather thin, quick, active, nervous and irritable. It suits the gouty and haemorrhoidal patients. The complexion looks muddy and the whites of the eyes are yellow and the urine is scanty and high coloured

NATRUM MUR : The patient requiring this remedy is sad, and hopeless about the future, easily angered and consolation aggravates the symptoms. There is weakness and prematurely aged look. Patient sheds floods of tears. With this remedy there is unpleasant recalling of past unpleasantness and grievances. His memory is poor, conversation disconnected, has hallucinations of hearing and delusions.

CIMICIFUGA : It is indicated in the depressed states. The patient is weak, depressed, suspicious people and objects appear strange and unnatural, the brain feels too large. This sensation of sadness settling over her is a great characteristic. There is always a feeling as if something is about to happen. There is a tendency to suicide. Visions of rats and mice are sometimes seen. Delirium from drink or uterine troubles is an important indication for this remedy.

□□□

CHAPTER 50

Tetanus

Tetanus is a specific infectious disease caused by the exotoxin of tetanus bacilli, usually growing in necrosed tissues, absorbed by the motor end plates of the peripheral nerves, carried to the central nervous system and manifested as lockjaw and paroxysmal spasmodic contraction of other muscles.

Tetanus bacilli present in the soil especially one contaminated by faeces of a horse or of a similar animal, enters through some skin abrasions and remain localized at the site. These are thereafter removed by phagocytes but if any lacerated tissue is present, more so if contaminated by pyogenic bacteria, these multiply and manufacture a highly potent exotoxin which is absorbed through the motor nerve end-plates in the muscles carried to the motor cells of the central nervous system, the sensory ones not being affected.

The posterior root ganglia act as filter preventing the toxin from entering into the spinal cord, the anterior root is thus only affected.

The toxin is so powerful that 0.0005 mg. may cause death of a mouse. When the toxin reaches the cord and brain stem, it becomes fixed on the nerve cells: when this happens in lethal dose, antitoxin administered therapeutically does not give protection. The subjects of any age even new born infants. The incubation period is 2 to 14 days.

The toxin by acting on the motor nerve cells makes them extremely hypersensitive. The disease starts with increasing tonic spasm of the masseter. The jaws become fixed and mouth does not fully open and from involvement of the muscles of deglutition, swallowing becomes difficult. The muscles of the back of the neck, face, pharynx, and abdomen's spine and afterwards those of the limbs are affected: adductors of the thigh may be affected early.

When the disease has fully developed taking from 12 hrs. to one-week, any external stimulus, ever-gentle touch, strong light and noise, proves the most agonizing clonic and tonic contractions of nearly all the muscles of the body. The jaws are firmly closed, teeth clenched, the facial muscles contracted. Contraction of the frontalis and of the muscles at the angles of the mouth causes risus sardonicus. The neck and the abdomen stiff and the spine arched backward, forward or sideways. The limbs are also stiff. If left alone for the time being, slow partial relaxation takes place till the next spasm starts.

The tendon jerks are exaggerated and on scratching the sole of the foot for the plantar reflex, the knee is extended. The skin is bathed in sweats during and after the convulsive attack.

The pulse and respiratory rates are usually unaffected and the temperature is not often raised except in the state of convulsion when these are increased. The mind remains clear till the end. Blood shows a moderate degree of leucocytosis. The cerebrospinal fluid is clear but is often under pressure.

CEPHALIC TETANUS following wounds of the face, head and neck causes a severe type of the disease with convulsion dysphagia and paralysis of the facial muscles of one side and spasm of the muscles of the opposite side along with trismus and ocular palsy: often ends fatally.

LOCAL OR MODIFIED TETANUS: With a prolong incubation period even reaching 30 days, only the muscles in the neighbour hood of the infection are in spasm: this is common in persons who received prophylactic inoculation. This spasm may continue for weeks or months and then gradually disappears or may be followed by general spasm.

In a favorable case, the spasms are mild and tend to become progressively less and muscles relax during the interval. In an unfavorable case with involvement of many muscles, the spasm increases, temperature rises high and the urine contains acetone, albumin and cast.

The prognosis is unfavorable in children and in cases with short incubation period.

Death takes place from

i) muscular exhaustion and heart failure
ii) asphyxia from spasm of glottis.

The characteristic points of diagnosis are:

a) Previous history of street injury and soil contamination

b) Initial symptoms starting with trismus.

c) No complete muscular relaxation during the intervals of spasm.

d) Mind remains clear and

e) Fatal termination in a large number of cases.

Treatment is available in homoeopathy. A few important medicines are given below:

Homoeopathic Medicines

CICUTA VIROSA: A useful remedy in tetanoid convulsions, with sudden rigidity and jerkings followed by prostration. There is great oppression of breathing, locked jaw, opisthotonos renewed by touch. There are oesophageal spasms and a marked symptom is fixed eyes staring at one point. Spasms and cramps in muscles of nape of neck, and spasmodic drawing backward of head. Curved limbs cannot be straightened nor straight ones bent. Back bent backward like an arch, jerking, tearing in coccyx, especially during menses. Trismus; disposition to grind teeth. Sensation of internal chill.

NUX VOMICA : It has titanic convulsions with opisthotonos, distortion of eyes and face, with dsypnoea excited by any external impression. Respiratory spasm with blue cyanosed face and clear mind. Nux always seems to be out of tune; inharmonious spasmodic action. Arms and hands go to sleep. Paresis of arms with shocks. Legs numb; feel paralyzed; cramps in calves and soles. Cracking in knee joints during motion. Sensation of sudden loss of power of arms and legs in the morning.

CUPRUM METALLICUM : Face is pale, jerking, opisthotonos; patient loses consciousness with each spasm. Convulsions beginning in the fingers and toes, violent, contractive and intermittent pain. Jerking, twitching of muscles. Coldness of hands. Cramps in hands. Cramps in calves and soles. Clonic spasms, beginning in fingers and toes. Chorea brought on by fright. Movement and touch increase the pains. Bruised pain in brain and eyes on turning them. Purple red swelling of head, with convulsions.

STRAMONIUM : Tetanic convulsions, spasm of glottis and chest worse from light or touch. Sensation as if limbs were separated from body. Absence of pain and muscular mobility especially of muscles of expressions and of locomotion. Convulsion of upper extremities and of isolated groups of muscles. Chorea, spasms partial, constantly changing. Violent pain in left hip. Trembling, twitching of tendons, staggering gait.

HYDROCYANIC ACID : It is a very good remedy for tetanus. It produces a tonic spasm from its direct action on the spinal cord. It shows itself in the muscles of the face, jaws and back. There is trismus or locked jaw, risus sardonicus and impeded respiration, with lividity and frothing at the mouth; the rigidity is firm, the body is bent backwards, the attack is sudden, and there is less reflex excitability. Spasmodic constriction in larynx, feeling of suffocation, pain and tightness in chest. State of collapse. Jaws clenched in rigid spasm. Froths at mouth. Pale bluish lips.

PHYSOSTIGMA : Here the sensory nerves are irritable; there are titanic spasms, stiffness of spine and legs, alternate dilatation and contraction of pupils. Meningeal irritation, with rigidity of muscles. Tetanus and trismus. Depresses the motor and reflex activity of the cord and causes of loss of sensibility to pain, muscular weakness, followed by complete paralysis, although muscular contractility is not impaired. Spinal irritation, loss of motility, prostration with very sensitive vertebrae.

□□□

CHAPTER 51

Thyroid Gland

It is a small mass of tissue present on either side of the trachea or windpipe. It is a very important structure that helps in the metabolism of the body.

When the basal metabolism is below normal, a person tends to be slow in his movements. He feels cold more and may have marked dryness of the skin, along with constipation and a tendency to put on weight. His hair is dry, thin, and coarse and the skin appears dry, scaly and thickened. There may be puffiness in the face, especially around the eyes. The tongue is usually large, the pulse is slow and regular, and the patient often complains of vague pains in the back and stiffness in the joints.

Hypothyroidism: It is a condition that results from the insufficient amount of thyroid hormone in the body. The trouble may also develop from pituitary deficiency, but is more likely due to some inborn error of the thyroid gland. The change usually comes gradually and involves the patients personality and also his ability to think.

Hypothyroidism is seen in both sexes, but is more common in women. Most of these are overweight and may complain of heavy flow during menstruation. The heart is often enlarged, and there is high level of cholesterol in the blood stream.

Hyperthyroidism: It is also known as Grave's disease or thyrotoxicosis. It is a serious condition of the body, arising from too much activity of the thyroid gland. The increased amounts of thyroid hormone produced by the overactive gland will then raise the metabolic rate of the body.

It is mainly present in the age group of 20 -30 years of age. It is more frequent in males but is more dangerous in females. Violent emotions, fear, anger and grief are thought to be exciting causes. Prolonged lactation, or diarrhoea, excessive mental work is predisposing causes. Other important causes may include heredity, traumatism, physical strain, mental overwork, toxemias, and dysfunction of the internal glands especially the adrenals.

As a result of the tachycardia myocardial degeneration may result. The orbital adipose is increased; also an increase of blood and lymph in the orbit. The enlargement of thyroid is due to marked dilatation of its blood vessels, especially the arteries.

"It is a peculiar disease combining three characteristic conditions namely: protrusion of the eyeballs, enlargement of the thyroid gland and functional disturbances of the heart. The neurotic symptoms are the early to appear. The tremors, which are involuntary and fine, may number from 425 to 500 per minute.

Palpitation of the heart, which accompanies the tachycardia, is at first light but increases rapidly, usually brought on and always aggravated by mental excitement. The heart beat runs from 100 to 160. Symptoms of neurasthenia may be present. Great excitability, mental depression and melancholia are frequent symptoms.

Exopthalamus varies in different patients. Immobility of the upper lid, a white line is noticeable above and below the cornea and marked dryness of the membrane is the important eye symptoms. Abnormalities of the optic nerve are rare. Ulcers of the cornea may also occasionally occur. The arteries of the retina may pulsate with the heartbeat.

The skin symptoms are: slight rise of temperature, sometimes profuse sweating, urticaria, pruritis, in advanced cases oedema, especially of the ankles, frequent flushing of the face, epistaxis, vomiting and purging.

A patient with this disease is usually nervous, weak, sensitive to heat, sweats frequently, is overactive and often underweight, inspite of an increased appetite. The patient eats healthy but continues to lose weight because of the higher rate of metabolism in the body.

Homoeopathic Medicines

BELLADONNA : This remedy acts powerfully on the brain and nerves, on the heart and circulation, and on the eyes. The patient is excitable, worries over small things, is violent in emotions, the pulse is full, rapid, bounding, there is throbbing in the carotids, the temperature of the skin is increased, the skin may be moist or dry, the eyeballs are prominent, pain deep in the eyeballs, the pupils dilated, the mucous membrane dry, the lids stiff, swollen and dry;

occasionally the Belladonna patient will have some tremors. The patient is full blooded, blood pressure is raised. . Nausea and vomiting. Great thirst for cold water. Spasms of stomach. Vertigo with falling to left side or backwards. Sensitive to least contact. Much throbbing and heat. Headache from suppressed catarrhal flow. Pain worse light, noise, jar, lying down and in afternoon; better by pressure and semi erect posture.

FEERUM PHOS : It is especially suited to anaemic patients of nervous temperament. The face flushes a bright red colour. When the flush is gone the face is pale and the mucous membrane of the lips and mouth becomes pale. Pulse is rapid, full and soft. Heart suddenly bleeds itself into the blood vessels and as suddenly draws a reflex, leaving pallor of the surface. Eyelids feel dry and as if sand were under lid. The menses are too frequent and too profuse, bright red bleeding from the nose.

SPONGIA TOSTA : Mental excitement aggravates all the subjective symptoms of the Spongia. There is a feeling of constriction and dryness in the larynx. Patient is awakened suddenly after midnight with pain and suffocation, surging of heat into the chest as if it would force out upward, rapid and violent palpitation with dyspnoea, cannot lie down, hypertrophy of the heart, especially the right. There is itching, swelling and induration of glands, during the menses the patient wakens with suffocative spells. Exhaustion and heaviness of the body after slight exertion, with orgasm of blood to chest, face. Anxiety and difficult breathing. Rapid and violent palpitation with dsypnoea. Feels best resting in horizontal position. Valvular insufficiency.

IODIUM : Rapid metabolism, loss of flesh with great appetite. Hungry with much thirst. Better after eating. Great debility, the slightest motion causes perspiration. Iodium patient is exceedingly thin; dark complexioned with enlarged lymphatic glands, has voracious appetite but gets thin. Abnormal vasoconstriction, capillary congestion followed by oedema, ecchymosis, haemorrhage and nutritive disturbances are important symptoms. Weakness and loss of breathe on going upstairs. Heart feels squeezed. Myocarditis, painful compression around heart. Feels as if squeezed by an iron band followed by great weakness and faintness. Palpitation from least exertion. Tachycardia. Skin is hot, dry and withered. Flushes of heat all over the body.

□□□

CHAPTER 52

Tonsillitis

At the back of the mouth on each side there are two small lymphoid organs known as tonsils. Normally they are about the size of a Lima bean, but they can become very larger if severely infected. The lingual tonsil is located at the back of the tongue close to other tonsils. There are two more lymphoid masses of tissue behind the soft palate known as adenoids. They make protective ring at the back of the nose & throat to keep infection from spreading throughout the body. Most of the germs enter through the mouth, nose and throat.

After becoming an adult the adenoids have largely disappeared. In childhood both the tonsils and adenoids may become very large. It makes swallowing painful and breathing difficult. In childhood large tonsils are common. The main reason of infection is due to certain types of streptococcus germs. Mouth breathing, nasal speech, a chronic cough are caused by the enlarged adenoids. The patient may also have halitosis or bad breath.

Causes of the first class are *predisposing*, i.e., the tubercular or rheumatic diathesis, and exciting, i.e. taking cold and bad hygienic conditions. Causes of the 2nd stage are the same as of first but plus the infectious diseases such as diphtheria, scarlet fever etc. This disease is more common between the ages of 10 and 25. Chronic tonsils may be of any form or all of the three forms. Heredity should be added to causes in all forms.

The changes may vary from any other portion of the glands, such as ulceration, pus, vitiated secretions, hypertrophy and atrophy or a simple inflammation of the covering membrane to complete destruction of that membrane.

Acute tonsillitis : Attack comes on suddenly with chills, fever, headache, weakness and pains in various parts of the body. There is a difficulty in swallowing due to sore throat. The tonsils appear red, large and spotted yellowish white pus, which may be seen oozing from the crypts or cavities on the surface of the tonsils. The inflammation of acute tonsillitis may spread to the middle ear, causing deafness, mastoditis and pain full lymph glands in the neck if not treated timely.

The presence of streptococcus germs within the throat may result in rheumatic fever, rheumatic heart disease and Bright's disease of the kidneys. Tonsils should always be treated seriously.

Symptoms may vary greatly, such as chilly sensations or marked chill; arrest of secretions, dry mouth and fauces, the secretions may become very profuse; surface may be covered with creamy pus; slight swelling of the local lymphatic; epithical cells & different micrococci in the form of a cheesy mass may fill crypts; calcareous degeneration occurs and deposits of lime may be found in the lacunae; the glands may become enlarged, then suppurate, during which we may have all the symptoms of sepsis; hypotrophy with mouth breathing, etc. finally atrophy may follow.

Homoeopathic Medicines

BARYTA CARBONICA : This remedy is the most prominent for Acute Tonsillitis. It has been of unfailing efficacy. Its use especially when the trouble is in the parenchyma of the glands and suppuration follows its use. It removes the predisposition to attack Belladonna is more superficial and Apis has oedema. It is useful where every cold settles in the tonsils. Especially in children who have chronic enlargement of those glands. The main use of Baryta has been, however in chronic enlargement of the tonsils. In a tendency to tonsillitis to scrofulous children with enlargement of other glands it will be found useful. Belladonna seems to have an affinity for right side. Children are backward and bashful requiring Baryta.

CALCAREA PHOSPHORICA : In chronic enlargement of the tonsils in strumous children this remedy stands well in typical Calcarea cases. The tonsils are flabby, pale; there is a chronic follicular inflammation and impaired hearing. Suffocative cough better by lying down. Hoarseness. Pain through lower left lung. Cannot open mouth without pain. Complaints during teething. Adenoid growths.

BELLADONNA : It is one of the most important medicines for right-sided tonsillitis. There is redness and swelling. The neck is swollen and stiff externally, ulcers form rapidly. In the acute paroxysms of the chronic form Belladonna is very useful. Throat is dry as if glazed. Throat feels constricted. Difficulty in swallowing anything worse liquids. Spasms in throat.

❑❑❑

CHAPTER 53

Varicose Veins

As the blood returns to the heart it passes through special thin walled vessels called veins. Unlike the tough strong arteries, these vessels are easily distended. One can demonstrate by pressing the finger on a vein on the back of hand and watching it swell as the blood builds up behind it. Blood flowing from the head and upper chest flows downward toward the heart. On the other hand, blood coming from the lower extremities must flow upward. To make this possible nature has provided valves in the veins so that the blood can flow only toward the heart, never in the other direction.

In human beings there are two sets of veins. The deeper veins are located within the muscles where they are given good support. But the veins on the surface just under the skin have little support and are easily damaged. These surface veins are often subject to inflammation or phlebitis.

In some people the veins in the legs are weak and may swell easily. Varicose veins, seems to run in families. Anything that increases the pressure in the pelvis or abdomen may slow the flow of blood back to the heart from the lower extremities. One frequent cause of varicose veins is pregnancy; other is obesity. Anything that increases the pressure within the veins of the legs and thighs may weaken or break down the little valves, so that the veins become enlarged and the blood does not finds its way back to the heart as it should.

Varicose veins are ugly, and sometimes they are dangerous. A blood clot forming within a greatly dilated vein may break off and travel to the heart and lungs. This serious condition, known as pulmonary embolism, may actually cause death. Serious hemorrhage may occur if a large varicose vein is torn open or cut. Some people have actually bleed to death, not knowing what to do in such emergency. Steady pressure over the bleeding point will usually control the bleeding. But one should avoid such a danger by having the veins properly treated.

People with varicose veins first note swelling along the course of the veins, followed by muscle cramps and a tired feeling in the legs behind the knees. In some cases the skin over the lower part of the leg may break down, forming a large, ugly ulcer, which is often painful, especially when thrombophlebitis develops in the leg.

To avoid further trouble one should not wear any elastic bands around the legs. Varicose ulcers need special care. The patient should rest in bed, with the legs elevated so that the heel is higher than the knee. Keeping the leg elevated will reduce the swelling by helping the blood return to the heart.

Homoeopathy has a very good treatment for varicose veins, which can save the patient from surgery. Indicated medicines are given below:

Homoeopathic Medicines

ARSENIC ALB : There is trembling, twitching, spasms, weakness, heaviness and easiness in the extremities. Cramps in calves. Swelling of feet. Burning pains. Ulcers in heel. Paralysis of lower limbs with atrophy. Skin is itching, burning, swelling; oedema, eruption, popular, dry, rough, scaly worse cold and scratching. Gangrenous inflammations. Ulcers with offensive discharge. Patients conditions are worse in wet weather, after midnight, from cold, cold drinks or food. Better from heat, from head elevated and from warm drinks. It irritates, inflames, and destroys all tissues. It acts rapidly and violently. Burning is the ranking sensation. Debility, exhaustion and restlessness with nightly aggravation are the leading indications for this remedy. Great exhaustion after the slight exertion. Burning pains. Unquenchable thirst for small quantities of water at small intervals.

FLOURIC ACID : It acts especially upon lower tissues, and indicated in deep, destructive processes, bedsores, ulcerations, varicose veins, and ulcers. Complaints of old age, or the prematurely aged, with weak, distended blood vessels. Ulcers; red edges and vesicles. Decubitis; worse warmth. Itching of cicatrices. Feels as if burning vapor were emitted from pores. Profuse, sour, offensive perspiration. Dropsy of limbs in old feeble constitutions. Atony of capillary and venous system. Tissues bloated. Patient is worse from warmth, in the morning, warm drinks. Better by cold, while walking.

CALCAREA FLOUR : It is a powerful tissue remedy for hard, stony glands, varicose and enlarged veins and malnutrition of bones. Induration threatening suppuration. It is a useful remedy after operations; the tendency to adhesions is reduced. Whitlow, indolent, fistulous ulcers, secreting thick, yellow pus. Hard elevated edges of ulcers, surrounding skin purple and swollen. Indurations of stony hardness. Swellings or indurated enlargements having their seat in the fasciae and capsular ligaments of joints or in the tendons. Patient is worse during rest, changes of weather. Better by heat and warm applications.

CAUSTICUM : This medicine manifests its action mainly in chronic rheumatic, arthritic and paralytic affections, indicated by the tearing, drawing pains in the muscular and fibrous tissues, with deformities about the joints; progressive loss of the muscular strength. It is mostly suited to dark complexioned and rigid fibred persons. Restlessness at night, with tearing pains in joints and bones and faint like sinking of strength. Burning, rawness and soreness are characteristic symptoms of this remedy. Cannot walk without suffering. Unsteady walking and easily falling. Restless legs at night. Itching on dorsum of feet. Soreness in folds of skin, back of ears, between thighs. It is a very good medicine for old burns that do not get well and ill effects of burn.

LYCOPODIUM : Lycopodium is adapted more especially to ailments gradually developing functional powers, where the function of the liver is seriously disturbed. Atony. Malnutrition. Mild temperaments of lymphatic constitution, with catarrhal tendencies; older persons, where the skin shows yellowish spots, earthy complexion, uric acid diathesis, etc.; also precocious, weakly children. Symptoms characteristically run from right to left, act especially on right side of body, and are worse from 4 to 8 PM. Abscess beneath the skin worse warm applications. Skin becomes thick and indurated. Varicose veins, naevi, erectile tumours. Numbness, also drawing and tearing in limbs especially while at rest or at night. Profuse sweat of the feet. Sciatica worse right side. Cannot lie on painful side. Cramps in calves and toes at night in bed. Limbs go to sleep. Twitching and jerking.

STAPHYSGARIA : Muscles especially of calves, feel bruised. Backache; worse in morning before rising. Extremities feel beaten and painful. Joints stiff. Dull aching of nates extending to hip joint and small of back. Patient is worse from anger, grief, indignation, mortification, loss of fluids, sexual excesses and least touch on affected parts. Patient is better after breakfast, warmth and rest at night.

❑❑❑

CHAPTER 54

Whooping Cough

Whooping cough is highly infectious specific disease, commonly of children characterized by respiratory catarrh and a special type of cough with inspiratory laryngeal spasm producing a characteristic sound.

This is common in children below 6 years, females are attacked more. Atypical cases are sometimes seen in adolescents and adults.

The disease occurs sporadically and less commonly in epidemics. It occurs mostly in winters and spring and is more common in temperate areas. The causative organism is Haemophillus pertusis present in the upper respiratory tract, conveyed by the infected sputum droplets of the patient to the contacts during the earlier stages of catarrh and paroxysmal cough.

The incubation period is 7 to 15 days or more.

A moderate degree of laryngeal, tracheal and bronchial catarrh with peribroncholitis and acute localized emphysema of the lungs are often associated. The tracheobronchial glands are sometimes enlarged. Rarely the right heart may be dilated and there may be haemorrhage in the brain and the meninges.

The disease begins with a moderate degree of fever, coryza and acute bronchitis but the cough is more distressing: it tends to be in paroxysmal usually at night and is often followed by vomiting. This continues for 7 to 14 days. Fever now subsides but the paroxysms of cough increases and are more severe during night.

During the paroxysm, usually fever stops till now and the stage of whoop begins. The child often knows that the fit is coming. He tries to suppress it, often sits down or runs to the mother for help. The paroxysm starts with deep inspiration and rapid succession of short coughs allowing very little time for breathing so that the lungs get nearly emptied of air. The child is almost suffocated, opens out his mouth, protrudes the tongue, the eyes bulge out and he is cyanosed. The skin if often covered with sweats and the scalp and the neck veins distended. If he had recently taken any food it is vomited out. Suddenly the fits stop, relaxation follows, air is sucked with the characteristic whoop and often bead like masses of viscid mucus are expelled.

The paroxysms are sometimes spontaneous, but more often excited by some peripheral stimulus such as taking of food, exposure to chill, inhalation of irritating fumes or mental excitement. These are worse at night. In the early stages, fits are comparatively few: soon these increase in number, several of these come in succession leaving the child at the end thoroughly exhausted and bathed in sweats. In a severe case the face is flushed, eyelids are puffy and subconjunctival hemorrhage and sublingual ulcer are often produced and the paroxysm may last for 2 to 3 minutes. The number of paroxysm varies from 15 to 100 or over daily. This number is indicative of the severity of the infection. The paroxysms may continue from 3 weeks to 2 months, the intensity gradually lessens and convalescence follows.

An atypical mild case may however terminate in a week or 10 days; this is more common in adults. In them whoop may not be present; violent paroxysms of suffocating cough gives clue to diagnosis.

Physical signs in the lungs are scanty. The urine during the paroxysm shows a high percentage of uric acid.

Complications

i) *Bleeding from the nose or any part of the respiratory tract* : under the conjunctiva, in the retina, from the ears; occasionally under the skin and very rarely cerebral and meningeal hemorrhages

ii) Severe respiratory efforts may result in acute emphysema, interstitial emphysema, spontaneous pneumothorax and subsequently bronchiolectasis. Increased intrapulmonary pressure causes dilatation of the right heart. Asphyxia may cause convulsions, which sometimes are fatal.

iii) Loss of appetite and frequent vomiting causes progressive weakness and muscular wasting. Forcible protrusion of the tongue causes ulcer of the freanum. Excessive vomiting may cause dehydration especially if associated with diarrhoea.

iv) Constitutional disturbances that may follow are diffuse bronchitis. As after complication sometimes-pulmonary tuberculosis may follow or unresolved pneumonia may cause pulmonary fibrosis, rarely enterocolitis, polyneuritis and albuminuria, otitis media is fairly common.

The child is segregated for at least four weeks and a plenty of fresh air and light is allowed. Powerful reflex stimuli as overloading of the stomach, cold draught, crying or any other mental excitation are avoided.

Homoeopathic treatment for whooping cough is given below:

Homoeopathic Medicines

DROSERA : There is barking cough in frequent paroxysms as to prevent the catching of the breathe; worse in evening. All efforts to raise the phlegm end in retching and vomiting. The attacks are especially worse after midnight: the child holds its epigastrium while coughing. The Drosera child cries a great deal. It is the most useful drug in whooping cough than any other remedy. Cough very deep and hoarse. Yellow expectoration, with bleeding from nose and mouth. Rough, scraping sensation deep in the fauces and soft palate. Sensation as if crumbs were in the throat, of feather in larynx. Harassing and titillating cough in children- not all through the day but commences as soon as the head touches the pillow at night. Asthma when talking, with contraction of the throat at every word utter.

CUPRUM : In whooping cough accompanied with convulsions or when the paroxysms are long and interrupted. Spasms of the flexor muscles predominate. The cough is very violent and threatens suffocation. The patient cough up a tough, gelatinous mucus there is much rattling in the chest, and the face and lips are bluish. A great characteristic of the remedy is the relief from a swallow of cold water. Suffocative attacks, worse 3 a.m. spasm and constriction of chest. Spasm of the glottis. Dsypnoea with epigastric uneasiness.

BELLADONNA : In sudden violent paroxysms of whooping cough, without any expectoration and the symptoms of cerebral congestion are found in-patient. Epistaxis may accompany and the patient is worse at night. It is suitable in the beginning of the disease or later when there is fever. Attacks of cough terminate by sneezing. A tickling in the throat excites the cough. Retching and vomiting and pain in the stomach are prominent symptoms. The child grasps at the throat and clings to its mother as if frightened. The patient is drowsy, the patient does not sleep. Cough is spasmodic and the child cries after each paroxysm. Larynx feel sore. Cheyne-strokes breathing. Cough with pain in left hip. Barking cough, whooping cough, with pain in stomach before attack, with expectoration of blood. Larynx very painful. Stitches in chest when coughing. Respiration oppressed, quick, unequal.

IPECACUAHANA : convulsive cough, where the child stiffens out and becomes pale and loses its breathe, great nausea and relief from vomiting. A gagging cough is a good indication. The discharge of mucus is copious and tenacious and the patient is very weak after the attacks. Violent shattering coughs following each other in quick succession, not permitting recovery of breathe. The child is limp and weak. And there is free perspiration. There is great anxiety and weight about the chest; sudden wheezing, dsypnoea, threatening suffocation, aggravated by motion, the cough causes gagging and vomiting. The cough is constant, the chest seems full of phlegm yet nothing is expectorated and the extremities are covered with cold perspiration. The expiration is difficult; vomiting when it occurs is apt to relieve the attack. Yearly attacks of difficult shortness of breathing.

ANTIMONIUM TART : With this remedy the child is worse when excited or angry, or when eating; the cough culminates in vomiting of mucus and food. There is much rattling of mucus in the chest but the expectoration is slight. The child will be irritable and cross, and will cry when approached; the tongue will be white and weakness will be present. Diarrhea is present with great debility and depression of vital force and vomiting of dinner after midnight. It has a marked aggravation from warm drinks. With Antimonium tart there is great oppression of breathing, worse towards morning, compelling the patient to sit up to breathe. There are also sharp, stitching pains and high fever, perhaps it corresponds more to the catarrhal form than it does to the croupous form.

PART – III

HOMOEOPATHIC MATERIA MEDICA

CHAPTER 55

Aconitum Napellus

The word Aconite is derieved from ACONIS, a city of Bithynia (in Asia Minor). Also ACON means dart because the darts were poisoned with Aconite. Also, from Greek word ACONITUM means without soil, as this plant grows on a stony ground.

History and Authority: Master Hahnemann introduced it in homoeopathy in 1805.

A state of fear, anxiety; anguish of mind and body. Physical and mental restlessness, fright, is the most characteristic manifestation of Aconite. Acute sudden and violent invasion, with fever, call for it.

There is no medicine like Aconite Nap when a complaint is caused by exposure to dry cold weather or by fright or both. Aconite should be thought of as the first medicine in inflammation, inflammatory fevers, when an attack is acute, sudden and violent, when there is physical and mental restlessness and if the problem is recent and when all this is on account of exposure to dry cold weather. The parts of the body affected can be larynx, bronchi, pleura joints and even heart.

Thus in acute and sudden attacks of croup, bronchitis, pneumonia, pleurisy, rheumatism, tachycardia, use of Aconite Nap would be indicated.

It should be remembered that Aconite Nap is useful in the acute, first stage of congestion and inflammation. It is a short- acting remedy but does its job most effectively.

With inflammation, there is fever and fear. It is fear of death especially, but can also be fear of crossing a street, of social intercourse, of an impending disaster. If there is pain it would be intolerable, worse as the evening progresses and it would be accompanied by numbness, tingling. There is a sensation as if small insects were crawling on the skin.

Aconite greatly helps in fever when the following symptoms are present: " heat with thirst; hard, full and frequent pulse; anxious, impatient, agony". (Dr. Hering). The patient kicks the clothes off, is worse lying on the left side, in warm room or with warm covering. The fever is acute, sudden, short and high. The skin is bright red. The patient feels very weak and suffers from typical Aconite Nap 'fear'. Evening chill with cold waves passing through the body.

In children there might be sudden congestion of the brain with intense fever. In Croup, when the child awakens frightened and has a dry, hoarse, croupy cough, Aconite Nap is an immediate cure.

Urine is scanty. Red, hot, painful. Burning in urethra. Urine suppressed. Profuse urination with profuse perspiration and diarrhoea. A newborn may not pass urine because it has suffered shock in birth. Give him a dose of Aconite Nap. The retention of urine would be relieved.

A bursting, throbbing headache on exposure to dry cold wind needs Aconite Nap. Sudden, violent with fear with anguish. Exposure to cold, raw wind causes neuralgic pains in the face. The pain is like hot wires running along either side of the face. There is a sensation of numbness, followed by pain, which is intense. Along the nerves, there is a feeling of crawling creeping ants. An exposure to dry cold wind may bring terrible toothache. Aconite would relive all these symptoms.

Coryza attended with violent headache requires Aconite Nap. It comes suddenly on exposure to dry cold. Coryza of rosy and chubby babies.

Aconite Nap immediately relieves a sudden, blood red inflammation of the eye on exposure to dry cold wind. The lids have swollen rapidly and cannot be opened easily. There is a feeling of a foreign body present in the eye.

Similarly Aconite Nap would relieve a throbbing, intense and cutting pain in the ear from exposure to dry cold winds. Children get such attacks often in the evening after returning from the play fields.

Aconite Nap immediately relieves violent cough from inflammation of the throat, which is dry, red, and burning and smarting in tonsils. Similar relief is possible if the larynx is inflamed.

Aconite Nap is supreme remedy for pneumonia. There is sudden and speedy inflammation of the viscera, of the pleura, of the lungs, of the mucous membrane lining. Besides, there is shortness of breath, oppressed breathing on least motion. Hoarse, dry, croupy, cough. The mucous membrane may ooze cherry red blood. The mucus might be white but it is heavily streaked with bright red blood.

In acute asthmatic attacks Aconite Nap comes as a God send. Alternate ipecac every half an hour till the attack subsides.

Tachycardia. Affections of the heart with pain in the left shoulder. Stitching pain in chest. Palpitation, with anxiety, fainting and tingling in fingers. Pulse full, hard, tense and bounding, sometimes intermits.

Sciatica with sensation of ice cold water poured along the course of nerves responds to Aconite Nap. Do not forget crawling sensation, fear and restlessness.

Shooting pain in limbs with numbness and a tingling sensation, icy coldness and insensibility of hands and feet, hot hands and cold feet, rheumatic inflammation of joints, which are very sensitive, red, shining, swollen, all due to exposure to dry cold air are ameliorated by Aconite Nap.

Vertigo on account of fright needs Aconite Nap. There is fainting, trembling. Fright may threaten abortion, may induce jaundice and make it chronic.

Gastric catarrh, a sharp, acute painful inflammation of the stomach, responds to Aconite. There is retching, vomit of blood, of bile and fear of death, anxiety and restlessness. All this could have resulted from exposure to dry cold.

Terrible, allergic, reactionary urticaria with thirst, heat and fear of death, is taken care of by Aconite Nap.

Coffea or Nux Vomica counteracts too much Aconite.

Sulphur is a chronic of Aconite Nap, that is, it completes a cure begin with Aconite Nap.

The patient is better by uncovering and in open air. The patient is worse in the evening for chest problems, by lying on the left side, in a warm room with warm covering, from music and from tobacco smoke.

□□□

CHAPTER 56

Arnica Montana

The name ARNICA is derived from ARNAKIS means lambskin due to the wooly appearance of the leaf.

MONTANA from Latin word MOUNTAINOUS from the place that is grows.

History and Authority: Hahnemann introduced it in homoeopathic practice in 1805.

The part used is the entire fresh plant, including root.

Arnica is one of the most frequently used remedies in the homoeopathic materia medica. We think of it whenever injury, however remote, appears to be the cause of the trouble. The injury may be recent or remote. It may be a blow or a contusion. The patient has a bruised, sore feeling all over. Any surface on which the body lies appears to be hard. Various limbs of the body ache as if these have been beaten. Arnica is the remedy in such cases.

The key word in the use of Arnica is "Trauma". Traumatic injuries respond very well to Arnica. Concussion, fracture of the skull with compression of the brain, drilling and extraction of the teeth, blows on the stomach and so on. The eyes feel sore and bruised after strenuous application. Fatigue comes on after hard work. Joints injured. Back injured resulting in lameness and sore feeling. A sprained ankle. Pain in tennis elbow. The bruised joint turns black. The skin around the eye turns black because of an injury. An infant undergoes trauma while being born. In all such cases Arnica renders relief, reduces pain and swelling and gives comfort. Trauma of grief, of sudden loss, financial or otherwise, is relieved by Arnica.

The patient is morose; does not wish to be physically touched; wants to be left to him. His body is sore. His mind is irritable, sad and fearful. He has fearful dreams. He goes into a stupor. He needs Arnica.

When a person suffers haemorrhage as a result of mechanical injuries, thinks of Arnica. Arnica should not be used externally in its pure form but internally it is the medicine. Use Arnica as a first aid remedy in cerebral haemorrahge. Also in bleeding from nose due to physical injury.

The skin can turn black anywhere on account of injury. Internally the mucous membrane bleeds easily. Arnica relieves the symptoms as well as the pain.

Arnica can be used as a healer and a preventive of sepsis before surgery of any type. It should be given in 1000 potency at least half an hour before the surgeon has to wield the knife. The healing process is speeded. Even after the surgery is over, Arnica 1000 should be administered once a day for at least a week to ensure a recovery free of complications. When you go for tooth extraction take Arnica 1000, in the same manner as above. (If bleeding does not stop after wards, Phosphorus 200 is also called for).

Arnica prevents pus formation, sepsis after injuries.

Patient desires for vinegar. Distaste for milk and meat. Canine hunger. Vomiting of blood. Pain in stomach during eating. Gases pass upward and downward. Pressure as from a stone.

Rheumatic lameness with joints lame, swollen and sore is alleviated by Arnica. Gout. Great fear of being touched or approached. Pain in the back and limbs, as if bruised or beaten. Sprained or dislocated feeling. Soreness after overexertion. Cannot walk erect, on account of bruised pain in pelvic region.

Arnica is useful when a person suffers angina pectoris (spasmodic choking and suffocating pain in the region of the heart). There is severe pain in the elbow of the left arm. The pulse is feeble and irregular. The breathing difficulty is distressing. The pain comes on account of insufficiency of oxygen or due to fatigue or both. This is an emergency situation when the patient must be made completely immobile and medicine administered as early as possible. Do not forget to consult a doctor without delay. But give Arnica 1000 immediately.

Over - work can make a person restless and sleepless. Once again Arnica helps. Comatose drowsiness; dreams of death, mutilated bodies, anxious and terrible. Horrors in the night. Involuntary stools during sleep.

Hoarseness in voice sometimes comes from overuse. Arnica gives relief. Acute tonsillitis, swelling of soft palate and uvula. Pneumonia approaching paralysis. Raw sore feeling in morning. Cough produced by weeping. Bloody expectoration. Whooping cough, child cries before coughing.

Arnica is a very good remedy for typhoid fever. Shivering over whole body. Heat and redness of head, with coldness of rest of body. Feet and hands cold, sweat comes in the night. Arnica is an excellent in acute as well as chronic problems.

The Patient is better when lying down and lying head down.

The Patient is worse when on motion, by least touch, in damp cold and heat.

Recommended potency : 200,1000 & above.

□□□

CHAPTER 57

Arsenic Album

It is a deep acting remedy on every organ and tissue. Its clear-cut characteristic symptoms amid correspondence to many severe types of diseases make its homoeopathic employment constant and certain. Its general symptoms often alone lead to its successful application.

Arsenic should be thought of in ailments from alcoholism, ptomaine poisoning, stings, dissecting wounds, chewing tobacco; ill effects from decayed food or animal matter; order of discharges is putrid: in complaints that return annually. Anemia and chlorosis. Degenerative changes. Gradual loss of weight from impaired nutrition. Reduces the refractive index of blood serum (also China and Ferr. Phos.) Maintains the system under the stress of malignancy regardless of location. Malarial cachexia. Septic infections and low vitality.

Arsenic Alb. is frequently used remedy in homoeopathy. The following indications are available in almost every problem, which Arsenic has to deal with:

1. Total debility.
2. Restlessness, mental as well as physical. The patient cannot stick to a place even if there is no discomfort. Sleepless but unable to sleep.
3. Irritable, Anxious. Sad Anxiety alternates with fear. Have suicidal tendencies.
4. An acute burning sensation, burning in the brain, in the inner head, in the throat or skin, in the lungs, in the breasts, in the stomach, in the bladder, in the vagina. As if somebody has lighted a fire. Nightly aggravation.

5. Burning is relieved by heat, by hot drinks.
6. Unquenchable thirst. But the patient can take only little water at a time.
7. Secretions related to Arsenic Alb are excoriating. The nose and the eyes become red. At times the odour is foul, odour of gangrene, of dying flesh, of a cadaver.
8. Advanced inflammation (unlike the first stage of Aconite inflammation).

Sensitiveness is a predominant feature in Arsenic cases. Sensitive to touch, to smell, and over - sensitivity of all the senses. The Arsenic patient is a fastidious person.

Extreme weakness is experienced in typhoid as well as asthma. The Arsenic patient is weak out of all proportion to the sickness.

An interesting observation about Arsenic patients is that they are always freezing, cannot get enough clothing to feel comfortable and warm and that they suffer tremendously in cold. Invalids are always chilly. The extremities of such patients are swollen.

In fevers of a typhoid character, Arsenic is one of the best remedies. Total prostration is noticed along with restlessness. The temperature goes high. Arsenic follows Rhus Tox and should be given in later stages of typhoid.

In intermittent fevers, such as malaria, Arsenic is very useful if other symptoms indicated in the first paragraph are present. Headache is periodic. Burning sensation is relieved by hot application. The lips are dry, parched and cracked. The patient has quenchable thirst, although he takes only a little water at a time. Cold food totally disagrees. The vomit can be of any kind, from water to mucus to bile to blood, even of coffee coloured substances.

In pneumonia, in the last stage of pneumonia of old people with gangrene, with foul smelling expectoration, Arsenic is very useful.

Use Arsenic where breathing is oppressed, where there is cough and frothy expectoration, where breathing out makes a wheezing sound, where the patient must sit up to breathe because his air passages are constricted, where asthma has followed pneumonia or chronic lung troubles have followed eczema.

The pain in the stomach is unbearable. It is worsened by least intake of food or drink, particularly, cold food or cold drink. There might be diarrhoea with black, bloody and horribly offensive stool. The stomach burns inside and hot drinks relieve this burning. The tongue is dry, brown or black. Arsenic is indicated in such cases.

Food poisoning cases get relief from Arsenic Alb. Poisoning can be from decayed food, animal matter, fruit cut and left in the open.

Arsenic is an excellent remedy in burning of the anus. Every stool burns as though there were burning coals in the rectum. Piles burn.

Arsenic is most effective in acute coryza. This patient is always taking cold in the nose, always sneezing from every change in weather. When profuse discharge of mucus excoriates the lips and wings of the nose, when there is incessant sneezing and when there is terrible sensation, use Arsenic. There is amelioration by hot application. (It may be advisable to start with Merc. Sol 200 in such cases and follows it up by Arsenic 200 if full relief dose not occur in a day. If both these fail, use Nat. Mur 200).

In the eyes, Arsenic relives intense photophobia with burning, acrid discharge, copious flow, ulcerated, red, granulated lids.

Eruptions on the genitals with burning, ulcers spreading in all directions, herpes of foreskin and of labia, at times with a little offensive discharge, indicate Arsenic Alb. Touch aggravates. The penis is swollen; scrotum swollen; labia swollen. Hard swelling. Burning. Stinging pain. Syphilis.

Arsenic is a palliative in cancers of mammae, of uterus.

Tremendous relief by use of Arsenic Alb. has been noticed in suppressed chronic eczema. The skin is dry and scaly, but almost always burning. Malignant pustules cover the surfaced. Arsenic also helps in ulcers with an offensive discharge, in oozing pitholes on the skin.

In Arsenic complaints a tendency to shrivel is noticed on the skin. It looks wrinkled, prematurely old (even in throat problems).

Arsenic is of great use in diabetic gangrene in extremities and in taking care of ulcers on heels. It is excellent for oozing ulcers which burn like fire and which have a blue-black base. Gangrene in internal organs needs Arsenic.

The patient is better: from raised head, from heat, from warm drinks and by sweat.

The patient is worse: after midnight, from cold, from cold food, cold drinks and from movement.

CHAPTER 58

Belladonna

The word Belladonna is derived from two Latin words Bella means fine or beautiful and Donna means lady. Its generic name 'ATROPA' comes from the Greek fate ATROPOS, 'THE INFLEXIBLE ONE'.

Think of Belladonna if you see a red surface because this medicine is associated with red, blood shot eyes, red, puffed face, red, swollen throat, red skin, which radiates heat. This redness indicates inflammation. Thus a large number of acute inflammatory diseases respond well to Belladonna.

Belladonna problems come on suddenly, with violence, run a regular course and then disappear as suddenly as they come.

When an inflammation is localized, Belladonna is the remedy in the first stage. Such inflammation comes suddenly, is red, painful and throbbing. This can be in the head, throat, breast or anywhere else in the body. This can be in the form of a carbuncle or a boil, on a hand or on a foot. Belladonna controls and aborts the problem in its first stage.

The Belladonna patient experiences heat, intense heat, violent heat. He suffers a burning sensation. If he has a sore throat, it is like coals on fire.

The Belladonna patient, like an Arsenic patient wants water in small quantities often.

Besides being red, the inflamed parts swell rapidly and are extremely sensitive to touch. Further, all over there is throbbing from congestion and inflammation. The head throbs with pain. The carotids throb. There is delirium, spasm, jerks and twitching. All with great violence.

Although the pain comes suddenly and goes suddenly, the patient is very sensitive to his suffering. This pain is worse from motion, worse from cold and worse from being shaken. Even if the body of the patient is slightly rocked by accident, the suffering aggravates.

Belladonna causes delirium, wild and terrible delirium wherein the patient imagines that he sees ghosts, hideous faces, animals and insects. The patient is violent.

Belladonna is the remedy for acute, destructive mania. The patient indulges in all sorts of violence. He has to be chained. His face and skin are red and hot and so is his head. But his hands and feet are cold as ice.

The Belladonna patient suffers from hallucinations, a host of visual illusions, fantastic illusions. He lives in a world of his own, oblivious to the surrounding realities. At the same time his senses are acute.

Belladonna has been called a remedy for the head. The blood rushes to the head and makes it hot. The face becomes bloody red, hot, swollen and shiny. The upper lip, the pupils of the eyes and the eyelids swell. In sunstroke, Belladonna and Glonoine run neck and neck. So also in congestive headaches. But while Glonoine cases are aggravated by heat, Belladonna is sensitive to cold.

Congestive headache responds to Belladonna very well and so does a neuralgic headache. There is a throbbing pain and the patient is worse on bending forwards and downwards or even lying down. Putting pressure in the head helps and so does a semi-erect posture. The patient experiences pulsation as if hammers are hitting the inside of the sore skull. The head feels enlarged with pressure from within outwards. Such a headache might be the result of an exposure to cold air or of suppressed catarrh, or of sunstroke.

If the patient has violent pain in the face, a throbbing pain, worse on the right side, worse from movement and when the face is radiating heat, the carotids are throbbing and when all these symptoms result from exposure to cold wind, Belladonna gives quick relief. (If the patient has suffered paralysis of the face from exposure to cold wind, Causticum would be the remedy). There is intolerable twitching. The face is bright red, gradually becoming purple and there might be fever. Erysipelas of the face needs Belladonna for these symptoms.

In conjunctivitis, when the conjunctiva is red, the eyes are swollen, protruding, dry, burning and fiery, Belladonna gives quick relief. The photophobia is intense. The pain in the eyes is intense. There is inflammation in the optic nerve and in the retina. The patient suffers orbital neuralgia. Suffering of the eyes is worse from movement of the eyes or from motion otherwise and from light.

There is nothing to replace Belladonna in the treatment of tonsils when they are violent red, swollen, painful, burning and dry. The throat feels constricted. Deglutition is difficult.

Belladonna is needed in inflammation of the larynx. There is a clutching, choking sensation. Rawness in the throat, smarting, scraping, little mucus, dry cough. Sudden attack of hoarseness. Voice changes key. Loss of voice is sudden. Spasm in larynx.

In the treatment of intolerable pain in the middle and external ear. Belladonna is an indispensable remedy. One dose of 1000 or 100000 gives immediate relief.

The same is true if there is a throbbing pain in the teeth and when there is a gumboil, which is red, painful and throbbing.

In problems from which children suffer, which come suddenly, without warning like sudden and intense heat or fever, Belladonna is useful. The child is hot in the skin; his face is red; he jumps in his sleep as if he might go into a spasm. The infant experiences convulsions, associated with cerebral congestion.

Pain, burning, discomfort and distension in the stomach respond very well to belladonna if the patient is sensitive to touch, aggravates with the slightest motion and is even sensitive to bed-clothes.

Haemorrhoids, which are violently painful, intensely red, greatly swollen and inflamed, burn and are sensitive to touch, respond very well to Belladonna.

In menstruation which is too early, too profuse and where the blood is bright red and hot, even foul- smelling, Belladonna gives relief. The dysmenorrhoea pain is like labour pains. The characteristic Belladonna pain comes suddenly, stays for a few moments and leaves suddenly.

In females, Belladonna takes care of constant, violent, bearing down sensation. It is worse on lying down and is relieved by standing (Sepia and Lillium Tigrinum have this bearing down, worse from standing; the patient has to sit down, cross legged, to support the internal organs.)

Belladonna cannot be forgotten in inflammatory rheumatism, when the joints are swollen, red, hot and sensitive. The inflammation comes from sudden exposure and localizes itself. Even the slightest motion aggravates as in the case of Bryonia. The cramps are violent. Dr. J.T.Kent describes the sensitivity of a belladonna patient thus: "Belladonna is so sensitive in parts that the motions of talking are painful, in the sore spots."

Belladonna is of no help in a continuous fever like typhoid.

Recommended potency: 200, 1000,1000.

In acute cases, repeat 200 frequently.

The patient is Better: By pressure on head, In semi -erect posture, Rest.

The patient is worse : From motion. From being shaken. From a jar, from cold, Bending forward, downward, lying down, on the right side of the face and from light.

□□□

CHAPTER 59

Bryonia Alba

The word BRYONIA means growing rapidly, as the stem grows rapidly.

ALBA, from Latin word ALBUS means white as the roots and flowers are yellowish or white.

Bryonia affects especially the constitution of a robust, firm fiber and dark complexion, with tendency to leanness and irritability. It prefers the right side, the evening, and open air. Warm weather after cold days, to manifest its action most markedly. Bryonia acts on all serous membranes and the viscera they contain.

Bryonia gives remarkable relief in muscular pain, which aggravates on motion, in the treatment of bronchitis and inflammatory and congestive headache.

The character of the pain is "Stitching and tearing". An interesting feature of Bryonia pain is that patient feels better, ameliorated if pressure is applied to the painful part. The patient is comfortable when lying on the painful side.

Whatever is the name of the disease, if there is an increase in discomfort by movement and relief comes by standing still. Bryonia is indicated. That is why, besides its utility in aches in every muscle of the body. Bryonia has been found to be of great help in bronchitis and in a bursting headache, where it appears that the head would split open, headache, which increases by stooping or even by the winking of an eye.

The patient for whom Bryonia is indicated is exceedingly irritable because he does not like to stir. His movements increase his problems.

The mucous surfaces of a Bryonia patient are excessively dry, lack secretion. The lips are parched, dry and cracked. The stool is hard and dry as if burnt. The Bryonia dryness leads to excessive thirst, which can be quenched by large intakes of cold water.

As indicated above, an excellent result is obtained from Bryonia in stitching muscular pain, which increases on movement. Its particular influence for improvements seen when the knees are stiff and painful. The feet are swollen. The joints are red, swollen and hot. There is inflammation in rheumatism.

Bryonia is extremely well indicated when the neck is stiff and painful. Bryonia relieves similarly stiffness and pain in the small of the back, worse on movement.

The pain in Bryonia is persistent and its severity increases gradually (as against this, Aconite pain comes with violence and Belladonna pain with suddenness). That is why, in rheumatic pain, which comes with gradually increasing severity, wherein one joint after another gets involved and wherein quite a few joints are inflamed with pain and discomfort, Bryonia is indicated. The body parts grow hot and inflamed. The pain always increases on motion. For sheer self-preservation, such a person would be languid, dry and irritable. Even waking up in the morning, which means movement, is bothersome.

For bronchitis Bryonia is a remedy par excellence. The trachea and the lungs are infected. There is violent cough, worse on movement. On coughing there is pain in the chest, severe pain, stitching and tearing. The cough is dry and suffocating. There is not much mucus inside. Think of Pulsatilla also if, at times, greenish, yellow mucus is expectorated in bronchitis. When there is loose cough with soreness, Natrum Sulphuricum is the remedy. Stitching pain in the center of the ribs is a clear indication for Bryonia. Soreness in larynx and trachea. Cough dry, at night; must sit up, worse after eating or drinking. Difficult quick respiration worse every movement.

Bryonia headache comes early in the morning. Headache may be associated with indigestion, inflammatory and congestive complaints. Constipation headache. Obstinate. Persisting. There is relief on pressing the head by hand or tying it up. The pain is worse from every motion, even the winking motion of the eyes, from the movement of the lips while talking, from the effort put into thinking. It is so severe as if the skull would split open. There is pain in the eyes. Light aggravates, although the patient wants to open the windows and breathe fresh cool air. The headache is worse in a warm room. The mind is sluggish. The patient looks an imbecile.

Women often have pain in their breasts at menstrual period. The breasts are pale, hard, hot and painful. Bryonia is of great help in such cases. It is indicated in intermenstrual pain, with great abdominal and pelvic soreness. Menses come early and are worse on motion. There is a copious flow of blood.

Nausea and faintness when rising up. Thirst for large quantities of water at long intervals. Stomach sensitive to touch. Pressure in stomach after eating as of a stone. Dyspeptic ailments during summer heat. Tenderness of abdominal walls. Constipation, stools hard, dry as if burnt, seem too large. Stools brown, thick, bloody, worse in the morning, from moving, on hot weather.

The patient is better : At rest, Lying on painful side, from pressure - firm and strong, from cold air, cool application, by free perspiration.

The patient is worse : By any motion, in warm weather, warm room (Dizziness in a warm room). Too much clothing, eating, in the morning, Slight touch, on exertion; sitting up, if visitors come.

CHAPTER 60

Cactus Grandiflorus

The name CACTUS was originally given by Theophrastus, to a spiny plant of Sicily in Italy.

Act on circular muscular fibres, hence constrictions. It is the heart and arteries especially that at once respond to the influence of Cactus, producing very characteristic constrictions as of an iron band. This sensation is found in various places, oesophagus, bladder, etc. The mental symptoms produced correspond to those found when there are heart affections, sadness and melancholy. Haemorrhage, constrictions, periodicity, and spasmodic pains. Whole body feels as if caged, each wire being twisted tighter. Atheromatous arteries and weak heart. Congestion; irregular distribution of blood. Favors formation of clots speedily. Great periodicity. Toxic goiter with cardiac symptoms. Cactus is pulseless, painting and prostrated.

We use Cactus for constriction of the heart. It feels as if an iron band were preventing the normal movement of the heart. The pain is worse when the patient is lying on the left side.

Cactus has four leading indications, viz. haemorrhage, constriction, periodicity and spasmodic pain. The whole body feels as if it is caged, with each wire being twisted tighter.

In case of heart problems, there is a fluttering and palpitation of the heart, an irregularity in the action of the heart. The patient suffers from endocarditis, an inflammation of the layer of the epithelial cells which lines the cavities of the heart. There may be mitrial insufficiency with palpitation. There may be swelling of the left hand, of the left leg and foot. The left arm is numb. The circulation of the blood is spasmodic, irregular.

For heart problems cactus acts best in incipient cardiac incompetence. Cactus would relieve the pain of angina pectoris where there is suffocation, cold sweat and a constriction like that of an iron band getting tighter and tighter. Pain shoots down left arm.

The heart troubles, which are caused by inflammatory rheumatism, are relieved by Cactus and so is heamorrahge apparently coming in sympathy with the heart trouble. Pain in apex, shooting down left arm. Palpitation, with vertigo, dyspnoea, flatulence. Very acute pains and stitches in heart; pulse feeble, irregular quick, without strength. Endocardial murmurs, excessive impulse, enlarged ventricle. Low blood pressure.

Fever every day at same hour. Coldness in back and icy cold hands. Intermittent paroxysms about mid day (11 a.m.) accompanied by haemorrhages. Coldness predominates, cold sweat, with great anguish. Persistent subnormal temperature.

Sensation as of a weight on vertex. Right sided pulsating pain. Congestive headache. Blood vessels to the heart distended.

Constriction, pulsation, or heaviness in stomach. Vomiting of blood. Hard black stools. Sensation of great weight in stomach.

Cactus is a useful remedy in acute inflammatory rheumatism. Here too, there would be a feeling of constriction with spasm.

Constriction is a leading indication in the use of Cactus. But it need be confined to the heart. Cactus constriction, which is felt like a spasm, can be in the head, above the chest, in the diaphragm and all over the abdomen. There is constriction on the scalp, of the skin which grows tighter and tighter. It can be in the throat, in the oesophagus, wirer it causes a spasm and prevents the food going down. It can be in the vagina causing vaginismus, which prevents coitus in the uterus there are, violent cramps. Constriction in the bladder or rectum needs Cactus.

The pain in Cactus is violent, clutching and constricting. Screaming with pain is common in Cactus. The patient is compelled to cry out. He cannot stand the pain. Because of the intensity of the suffering the patient is fearful and distressed. A typical Cactus case would have total numbness of the left arm, along with a history of rheumatism. The left arm has a tingling and a crawling sensation. The face is flushed bright red, later becoming blue; the lips turn blue.

With the constriction of the heart comes constriction around neck, choking of the neck as from a tight collar.

Constriction of the neck of the bladder causes retention of urine. There is blood in the urine; blood with stool, blood, which clots, Cactus is indicated.

Constriction of the anus is looked after by Cactus. There is severe constipation, usually in connection with haemorrhoids.

Profuse bleeding from nose. Fluent coryza.

Sleepless on account of pulsation in different parts of body. Frightful dreams.

Cactus is useful in right - sided pain in the facial nerves.

Cactus helps in cases of persistent sub- normal temperature.

Oedema of hands and feet. Hands soft; feet enlarged. Numbness of left arm. Icy cold hands. Restless legs.

Palpitation day or night worse when walking and lying on left side and on approach of menses.

Fear of death; believes the disease is incurable.

Recommended potency:

1. Mother tincture most of the time. 10 drops in water, 4 times a day.
2. 30 in nervous palpitation.

The patient is better: in open air.

The patient is worse: Lying on the left side

❑❑❑

CHAPTER 61

Calcarea Carb

This great Hahnemannian antipsoric is a constitutional remedy. Its chief action is on the glands, skin and bones. Increased general and local perspiration, swelling of glands, scrofulous and rachitic conditions generally offer numerous opportunities for the application of Calcarea. A jaded state, mental or physical, due to overwork. Persons of scrofulous type, who take cold easily, with increased mucous secretion, children who grow fat, are large bellied, with large head, pale skin, chalky look, affections caused by working in water. Children crave eggs and eat dirt and other indigestible things; are prone to diarrhoea. Calcarea patient is fat, fair, flabby and perspiring.

In cases of deficient or irregular bone development, deformed extremities, a crooked spine, a softening of the bone, Calcarea Carb comes handy. While the Sulphur patient might be usually thin, lean and wiry, the Calcarea patient might be obese. But like Sulphur, Calcarea carb helps in easy relapses, interrupted convalescence.

Mentally if the patient is interested only in trivia, little things, is unable to perform sustained mental operations, gets tired from mental work, and is easily dominated by others, Calcarea carb is strongly indicated. Such a person is weary of life, hopeless, low spirited and melancholy. He is apprehensive. He is forgetful. Obstinate.

In sulphur the sensation of burning is a strong indication. On exactly the opposite side of the spectrum, Calcarea has a characteristic of coldness, icy coldness of internal and external parts of the head, coldness of the feet, of the legs. A sensation of coldness in the individual parts of the body as well as a feeling of general coldness always indicates the use of Calcarea Carb.

A very important symptom for the use of Calcarea Carb is profuse sweat on the head of a large - headed child. Of course, sweating can come in anyone and Calcarea is indicated. This sweating occurs in connection with a number of debilitating diseases. In all such cases, the extremities of the patient feel cold. The knees are cold and swollen and the patient suffers cramps in the claves. There is rheumatic pain, sharp, sticking as if parts of the body have been twisted with a wrench. Tearing pain in muscles. Cold damp feet; feel as if damp stockings were worn. Sour foot sweat. Weakness of extremities. Burning of soles of feet. Sweat of hands.

Pain in the back as if sprained, can scarcely rise. Pain between shoulder blades. Rheumatism in lumbar region, weakness in small of back. Nape of neck stiff and rigid.

Idea crowding in her mind prevents sleep. Horrid visions when opening eyes. Starts at every noise; fears that she will go crazy. Drowsy in early part of evening. Frequent waking at night. Night terror. Dreams of the dead.

Calcarea Carb is useful in cases of pernicious anaemia.

Polyps in the nose, ear, bladder, urethra etc are greatly helped by Calcarea. The polyps in the ears bleed easily. An offensive odour emanates from the nose. The nostrils are sore and ulcerated. The mouth persistently tastes sour. Abscesses in deep muscles, in the neck, in the thighs or in the abdomen require Calcarea.

In old, lingering cases of nasal catarrh, Calcarea is useful. The patient gets up in the morning and blows out large, black and bloody lumps. The nasal discharge is thick, yellow and rusty in the daytime.

Calcarea Carb helps in spots and ulcers on the cornea. In chronic dilation of the pupils, it is useful after Sulphur.

Swelling of thyroid in goiter responds to Calcarea Carb.

In infections of the chest, where the patient spits blood, has prolonged cough and expectorates thick, yellow mucus, Calcarea Carb is needed. The patient is worse going upstairs. Suffocating spells, tightness, burning and soreness in chest. Chest very sensitive to touch, percussion or pressure. Desires fresh air. Tickling cough troublesome at night, dry and free expectoration in morning; cough when playing piano, or by eating. Extreme dsypnoea.

In case milk disagrees with a patient and he has sour eructation and sour vomiting, Calcarea Carb is useful. Such a patient does not like fats. He loses his appetite after putting in extra hours of work. Mentally he feels jaded.

Menstruation with vertigo, too early, too profuse, too long, with cold, damp feet or milky leucorrhoea indicates use of Calcarea carb. Very heavy sweating on external genitals is a leading indication. Cutting pains in uterus during menstruation. Milky leucorrhoea. Burning and itching of parts before and after menstruation; in little girls. Increased sexual desire; easy conception. Breasts tender and swollen before menses.

On the skin eruptions of minute red spots due to the escape of small amounts of blood, need Calcarea Carb.

Malnutrition is one of the disorders calling for this remedy. Tardy development of the bony tissues with lymphatic enlargements. Curvature of the bones, especially spine and long bones. Extremities deformed, crooked. Softening of the bones, fontanels remain open too long and skull very large.

There is a peculiar symptom of the appetite that has been verified- "Longing for eggs, particularly in children, in sickness or during convalescence. The stomach externally is swollen or seems distended. Diarrhoea is worse in the afternoon. The patient is better when constipated.

Calc carb is the chronic of Belladonna. When Belladonna has repeatedly helped in an acute condition, Calcarea Carb will cure and prevent a relapse.

Bryonia and Calcarea Carb are not compatible with each other.

Recommended potency: 30 and 200

The patient is better by lying on painful side, in dry climate and dry weather and by sneezing.

The patient is worse while ascending, in water, from washing, in moist air, wet weather, from mental or physical exertion, on a full moon night and by standing.

CHAPTER 62

Carbo Vegetabilis

The typical Carbo patient is sluggish, fat and lazy and has a tendency to have chronic complaints. Blood seems to stagnate in the capillaries, causing blueness, coldness and ecchymosis. Body becomes blue icy-cold. Bacteria find a rich soil in the nearly lifeless blood stream and sepsis and typhoidal state ensues. Weakness due to excessive diarrhoea, menstruation or other debilitating diseases. The patient may be almost lifeless, but the head is not, coldness, breathe cool, pulse imperceptible, oppressed and quickened respiration and must have air, must be fanned hard, must have all the windows open. The patient faints easily, are worn out must have fresh air. Haemorrhages from any mucous surface. Indicated for persons who have never fully recovered from the effects of some previous illness. General venous stasis, bluish skin, limbs cold.

Homoeopathy has converted even a wood charcoal into a lifesaver. In this system, if there is a medicine which can bring a patient back from the jaws of death, it is Carbo-veg. The patient has been transiting from sickness to sickness. He has never fully recovered. He lies motionless as if dead. His breathe is cold, his pulse intermittent and he has cold sweat on the limbs. Yet he needs a strong fan. He cannot get enough oxygen. His face turns blue. The skin is pale. He appears lifeless, although is head is hot. His digestion is so weak. Debilitating haemorrhages have occurred from mucous surfaces. It may be a state of collapse in cholera and typhoid. The blood is disintegrating or there is imperfect oxygenation. The body is ice-cold. Such a patient revives with Carbo-Veg.

According to Dr. Nash, Carbo-Veg may save a life "in the last stage of disease, with copious cold sweat, cold breath, cold tongue, voice lost."

All disorders of the stomach respond to Carbo-Veg. eructation, heaviness, fullness, and sleepiness: tense from flatulence, with pain; worse lying down. Eructation's after eating and drinking. Temporary relief from bleaching. Rancid, sour or putrid eructation, Water bash, asthmatic, breathing from flatulence. Nausea in the morning. Burning in stomach, extending to back and along spine. Contractive pain extending to chest, with distension of abdomen. Faint gone feeling in stomach, not relieved by eating. Crampy pains forcing patient to bend double. Distress comes on a half - hour after eating. Sensitiveness of epigastric region. Digestion slow: food putrefies before it digests.

We have found Carbo-Veg most useful in acidity. In flatulence with eructation and a feeling of heaviness, Carbo-Veg does wonders. There may be at times constrictive pain extending to the chest with distention of the abdomen. The pain in the chest is like burning from glowing coals. The acidity and flatulence are ameliorated by belching or by passing flatus.

Carbo-Veg is one of the best remedies for slow digestion, for aversion to milk, meat and fats. Nothing expresses its utility as the statement, "the simplest food disagrees". For digestion of fats where Pulsatilla fails, Carbo Veg succeeds.

Carbo-Veg is an effective medicine in curing ulceration of the stomach. There is burning in the stomach extending to the back and along the spine.

Carbo-Veg helps retracted gums, which bleed easily. There is pyorrhea. Brushing the teeth makes the gums bleed.

Massive haemorrhage is checked by Carbo-Veg. The bleeding may be from the lungs, from the uterus, from the bladder or any other mucous surface. The surface appears to be too weak and spongy to hold the blood.

Carbo-Veg is a remedy in septic conditions, after surgical operations and after shocks. It greatly helps where any little inflammation or congestion has become black or purple.

In old people, Carbo Veg relieves an asthmatic attack, which makes the skin blue.

In desperate cases of pneumonia, Carbo-Veg helps where Antim Tart has failed to help the patient in clearing his lungs of threatening mucus, when the face turns blue and weakness at times is leading to a paralysis. The sputum is foul smelling. The patient wants to be fanned. It is the 3rd stage of pneumonia.

Carbo Veg is an excellent medicine for varicose veins in pregnancy or otherwise, and for varicose ulcers. Very good for gangrene.

Dr. Kent has called Carbo-Veg a friend to the woman and a friend to her offspring. It helps women who grow weak from nursing. It prepares a woman well for confinement and looks after would be mother in her rundown condition. It helps to relieve nausea in pregnancy as well as reduce the enlargement of the veins of the lower limbs, which one comes across in the circumstances. Of course, it helps in the pregnant woman's offensive flatulence, if any.

In some women one period runs into another. This type of weakening menstruation with dark, oozing blood needs Carbo-Veg.

Carbo-Veg is indicated after surgical shock, when the patient goes into collapse and is in danger of dying from the shock of the operation. The inflammation has yet to set, but there is not enough strength for this to happen. The heart is weak. Carbo-Veg doses would strengthen and give life to the patient.

Mentally a Carbo-Veg patient is indifferent. The most horrible things do not affect him adversely; pleasant circumstances do not cheer him up. He is in confusion. He cannot think. He looks stupid and benumbed.

Carbo-Veg is indicated when there is internal burning and external coldness.

China and Carbo Veg are complementary, that is, these help the patient if used in alternation depending on the facts of his case.

Recommended potency : 200,1000.

Higher potencies in chronic cases.

The patient is better : From eructation, Fanning cold air.

The patient is worse : In the evening; at night, in open air, Taking fats, butter, and coffee, milk, in warm, damp weather.

❑❑❑

CHAPTER 63

Causticum

Manifests its action mainly in chronic rheumatic, arthritic and paralytic affections, indicated by the tearing, drawing pains in the muscular and fibrous tissues, with deformities about the joints; progressive loss of muscular strength, tendinous contractures. Broken down senile. In catarrhal affections of the air passages, seems to choose preferably dark - complexioned and rigid fibered persons. Restlessness at night, with tearing pains in joints and bones, and faint - like sinking of strength. This weakness progresses until we have gradually appearing paralysis. Local paralysis, vocal cords, muscles of deglutition, of tongue, eyelids, face, bladder and extremities. Children are slow to walk. The skin of Causticum person is of a dirty white sallow, with warts, especially on the face. Emaciations due to disease, worry etc. Burning, rawness and soreness are characteristic.

Causticum is indicated in the treatment of chronic rheumatism and paralysis accompanying it. Here, Causticum ranks with Rhus Tox and Sulphur.

In rheumatism, there is excessive deformity of the joints. These are enlarged and soft and the pain is worse in dry weather. Rheumatism has affected both the muscles as well as the joints. The pain is tearing and benumbing. It takes the life out of a patient. It stays in parts of the body for a long time. Causticum is of great help in the lightning - like pain of locomotor ataxia.

Besides deformities of the joints, there is a tearing pain in muscular tissues and progressive loss of muscular strength. The patient is restless at night. There is gradually appearing paralysis, a local paralysis of the vocal cords with loss of voice, of muscles in the oesophagus, of the tongue, of the eyelids, face bladder and extremities. Paralysis of single parts. Numbness loss of sensation in hands. Restless legs at night. Cracking and tension in knees; stiffness in hollow of knee.

Causticum paralysis is generally on the right side (Lachesis helps in the left side paralysis.

Causticum take care of stiffness and pain in the neck and the throat. The muscles feel as if these have been bound with ropes. The patient can scarcely move his head. There is a dull, drawing pain in the arms and hands, a drawing and tearing pain in the thighs, legs, knees and feet.

Causticum also helps in the left sided sciatica with numbness.

It also helps in contracted tendons, tendons that have been shortened, resulting in a temporary or permanent contraction. The limb is drawn up. The problem may appear in the forearm particularly.

Causticum is a chronic remedy, useful in diseases, which have come over a long time. It is needed in old, broken down constitutions.

A causticum patient is melancholy, a pessimist, has forebodings. He is unhappy, suspicious and distrustful.

Causticum is a remedy in stammering. It is also useful in paralysis of both the pharynx and oesophagus. Such a paralysis might sometimes come at the end of diphtheria.

Loss of voice comes from paresis of vocal cords. This may also come for catarrhal reasons. There is rawness in the respiratory tract, an irritation in the trachea and a dry hollow cough. Hoarseness with pain in chest. Expectoration scanty must be swallowed. Cough with pain in hip, especially left worse in evening; better drinking cold water. Pain in chest with palpitation. Difficulty of voice of singers and public speakers.

Causticum is very useful in deafness when simultaneously there is a roaring noise, a tinkling noise or a humming sound.

Causticum comes next to Thuja in the treatment of warts. Old warts on eyelids, eyebrows, nose; warts on face. It also helps in soreness in folds of the skin, between the thighs and at the back of the ears. The warts which Causticum treats are large, jagged, easily bleeding and on the tips of the fingers and the nose.

Do not forget Causticum in old burns which do not get well. It also helps in the treatment of results of burn.

Causticum takes care of involuntary passing of urine when the patient is coughing or blowing his nose or sneezing. Involuntary during first sleep at night; also from slightest excitement. Retention of urine after surgical operation. Loss of sensibility on passing urine.

In anal problems, Causticum cures very specific symptoms. There is constipation with frequent but unsuccessful desire to pass stool. When the patient strains, his face becomes red. He can pass stool easily when standing. Haemorrhoids are swollen. There is itching, burning, stinging, smarting, rawness and moisture. The piles are worse on walking.

In women, Causticum is useful in uterine inertia during labor. Menses ceases at night; flow during day. Leucorrhoea at night with great weakness.

Causticum is incompatible with Phosphorus.

Recommended potency : 30, 200.

In chronic cases, higher potencies used infrequently.

The patient is better in damp and cold weather, in warmth and in the heat of the bed.

The patient is worse in dry, cold winds, in clear fine weather and from motion in a carriage.

❑❑❑

CHAPTER 64

Chamomilla

The word **CHAMOMILA** is derived from **CHAMAEMELUM** and **MATRICARIA** from **MATRIX** means apple on the ground, because the plant grows to the ground and has an odour like that of apples. It has been used since long as a domestic remedy by the name chamomile.

The chief guiding symptoms belong to the mental and emotion group, which lead to this remedy in many forms of disease. Especially of frequent employment in diseases of children, where peevishness, restlessness, and colic give the needful indications. A disposition that is mild, calm and gentle; sluggish and constipated bowels contra-indicate Chamomilla.

Chamomilla is sensitive, irritable, thirsty, hot, and numb. Oversensitiveness from abuse of coffee and narcotics. Pains unendurable, associated with numbness night-sweats.

The child patient wants to be carried in the arms. His mood is very irritable and snappy. He does not know what he wants. He needs a dose of Chamomilla. Even in elders, the patient is cross, ugly, spiteful and snappish. He cannot bear others. He cannot bear pain. He wants things but on getting them throws them away. He is uncivil.

Ailments brought on by fits of anger require Chamomilla. The nature of the ailment matters not. Chamomilla cures bad effects of bad temper.

A very important indication of the use of Chamomilla is the patient's sensitiveness to pain. His pain is associated with numbness and night sweats. The pain is disproportionate to the severity of the sickness. A dose of Chamomilla 200 relieves.

Chamomilla relieves any pain, accompanied by numbness, which is unendurable, whether it is a neuralgic pain, pain after tooth extraction, a toothache, labour pains, stomach pain, lumbago or a rheumatic pain. In most of these cases the patient is cross, peevish, restless and difficult to please.

Numbness with pain indicates Chamomilla more than anything else. This pain is aggravated by heat but is not relieved by cold (which is the case with Pulsatilla.).

Chamomilla is frequently used in the case of children suffering from dentition diarrhoea. The stool is hot green, slimy. It has white and yellow mucus, which looks like chopped eggs and spinach.

Violent rheumatic pain may drive the patient out of bed at night, compel him to walk about. There is excessive uneasiness and anxiety. Even in the abdomen there may be tearing pain. The pain being excessive, the sensitive patient would loose sleep. These indications require Chamomilla.

Chamomilla gives relief in earache when the pain, on account of swelling and heat, drives the patient mad. Stitching pain. Ears feel stopped

An interesting cure achieved by Chamomilla is the case of burning sole at night. The patient wants to put his feet out of bed. He gets comfort that way.

One cheek red and hot, the other pale and cold. Stitches in jaw extending to inner ear and teeth. Toothache worse after warm drink; worse after coffee at night.

Child wants many things, which he refuses again. Piteous moaning because he cannot have what he wants. Child can only be quieted when carried about and petted constantly. Impatient; intolerant of being spoken to or interrupted; extremely sensitive to every pain; always complaining. Complaints from anger and vexation. Mental calmness contraindicates Chamomilla. Peevish child: Chamomilla is used more frequently in the sickness of children than of adults. The child is peevish restless and has colic. His pain is intolerable.

Eructation foul. Nausea after coffee. Sweats after eating or drinking. Aversion to warm drinks. Tongue yellow; taste bitter. Bilious vomiting. Acid rising regurgitation of food. Pressive gastralgia, as from a stone. Distended. Griping in region of navel, and pain in small of back. Flatulent colic, after anger, with red cheeks and hot perspiration.

Hot, green, watery, fetid, slimy, with colic. Chopped white and yellow mucus like chopped eggs and spinach. Soreness of anus. Diarrhoea during dentition. Haemorrhoids, with painful fissures.

Uterine haemorrhages. Profuse discharge of clotted dark blood, with labor like pains. Labor pains spasmodic; press upward. Patient intolerant of pain. Nipples inflamed tender to touch. Infants breast tender. Yellow acrid leucorrhoea.

Violent rheumatic pains drive him out of bed at night; compelled to walk about. Burning of soles at night. Pain in ankles in the afternoon. Nightly paralytic loss of power in the feet, unable to step on them. The patient often very sensitive to cold, and cold air brings on troubles for which this remedy is specific.

Another condition, which is met by this remedy, is restlessness and sleeplessness. The patient is maddened; driven to desperation under Chamomilla; does not care whether she dies or not, had rather die than suffer. The sleeplessness of Chamomilla patient is owing to the pain and excessive nerve sensibility and this remedy procures sleep by overcoming these troubles, which make the patient sleepless.

Recommended potency: 30 for children. 30 and 200 for adults.

The patient is better from being carried and in warm and wet weather.

The patient is worse by heat, anger, by exposure to fresh air, during nighttime in bed, in winter and in cold weather.

□□□

CHAPTER 65

Cinchona Officinalis (China)

CINCHON, a place where the Countess Ann, a wife of the 4th Count of CINCHON lived. She was cured by tertian fever in 1638 by the use of cinchona bark. Its virtues were made known to Europe in 1640. The botanists identified it in 1717. This drug shows the pathway for the establishment of homoeopathy.

The key word in the prescribing of China is 'debility' or weakness caused by excessive loss of blood or other fluids from the body, through nursing or salivation or excessive and bloody leucorrhoea, menstruation or long-continuing diarrhoea or through profuse pus formation or after an attack of influenza. There may be haemorrhages from the wounds, the lungs, the bowels or from the nose, a sudden depletion leading to fainting, loss of sight, ringing in the ears or to an over all weakness of the body. China acts as a marvelous remedy in such cases. The dose should be frequently repeated in 200 potency.

The debility of a China patient is partly indicated by darkness before the eyes, ringing sounds in the ears and fainting on the slightest provocation. His face is pale, sallow, eyes are sunken and he sweats easily on least motion or labor. There is loss of memory. The mind is weak and unable to think. The patient chooses wrong words and expressions. In Dr. J.T. Kent's words, he is 'apathetic, indifferent, low spirited, silent, disinclined to think'. In women, haemorrahges from uterus followed by sleeplessness night after night. They feel dizzy and faint. The patient is averse to exercise, to work.

Periodicity in the onset of disease is an important indication for the use of China. The pain comes with regularity at a given time each day. It increases sharply at midnight. That is why China has been found useful in intermittent fevers coming at fixed intervals with well-marked stages. Thirst precedes the chill, which generally comes in the forenoon. The night sweats are so profuse as to cause extreme debility.

A China patient bleeds easily. The bleeding may be from any surface of the body, from the nose, from the throat, from the lungs, or from the uterus. Inflammation of the bleeding part of the body follows rapidly and the affected area turns black. Convulsions come in the midst of bleeding, such as confinement. Dropsy follows loss of blood.

In cases as if the skull would burst with headache. There is an intense throbbing of carotids. The patient experiences vertigo while walking. China helps in such cases.

There is nothing like China where the abdomen is bloated likes a tent. Flatulence causes colic and it is all over. There is no relief on belching or on passing wind. Movement gives comfort, however digestion is slow but the hunger is acute at meal times.

The stool is watery, light coloured, undigested, painless. The abdomen gurgles and rumbles. Flatus is discharged without relief. Such diarrhoea is common in children. There is aggravation at night. China is indicated.

In chronic liver trouble with pain in the right side, where the liver is enlarged, is hard and sensitive to touch, where the spleen is swollen, china brings relief. The China patient cannot bear the slightest touch. But hard pressure on the suffering part of the body gives him relief. The pain increases periodically. Suffering is worse by exposure to a draught of air.

For women, China is a blessing when the menstruation is profuse and painful. There is abnormal abdominal distention. She passes dark clots of blood. Even leucorrhoea is bloody. The menstruation quite often starts too early.

China is useful in typhoid and malaria only when periodicity is marked, night sweats are profuse and there is depletion of fluids. There is a shaking chill over the whole body. Aggravation at night. Free perspiration caused by every little exertion, especially on single parts. Hay fever, watery coryza, pain in temples.

Vomiting of undigested food. Slow digestion. Weight after eating. Ill effects of tea. Hungry without appetite. Darting pain crosswise in hypogastrium. Milk disagrees. Hungry longing for food, which lies undigested. Hiccoough. Bloated ness better by movement.

Undigested, frothy, yellow, painless worse at night, after meals, during hot weather, from fruit, milk beer. Passing of stool is difficult even when soft. The stools are also accompanied with large discharge of flatulence.

Inflammatory rheumatic pain coming at a fixed time is relieved by China. Pains in limbs and joints as if sprained; worse slight touch, hard pressure relieves. Joints swollen, very sensitive, with dread of open air. Averse to exercise; sensitive to touch. Weariness of joints; worse mornings and when sitting. Knife like pains around back.

Irregular with weak rapid beats followed by strong, hard beats. Suffocative attacks, syncope, anaemia and dropsy.

Influenza with debility. Cannot breath with head low. Labored slow respiration; constant choking. Suffocative catarrh, rattling in chest. Violent hacking cough after every meal. Haemorrhages from lungs. Dsypnoea, sharp pain in left lung. Asthma; worse damp weather.

Recommended potency is tincture to 30th potency.

Patient is better from bending double. Hard pressure, open air & warmth.

Patient is worse from slightest touch, draught of air, loss of vital fluids, at night & after eating.

□□□

CHAPTER 66

Gelsemium

The word *GELSEMIUM* is derived from Latin word *GELSIMINO* meaning jasmine and *SEMPERVIRENS* meaning ever green.

Gelsemium is one of the most effective remedies in the treatment of influenza where there is body pain, pain in the head at the base of the brain, that is, in the occiput, and where there are accompanying throat problems.

Mentally, the Gelsemium patient desires to be left alone in peace. He is torpid, sleepy and dreads movement. He is dull. He cannot think clearly or concentrate.

As indicated above, Gelsemium is one of the remedies used in the treatment of influenza where there is body pain, a feeling of chill going upwards in the spine and congestion on the occiput. The eyes burn and itch with great discomfort. The patient sneezes and experiences coolness at the root of the nose. There may be acute running nose with dull headache and fever. At times the nose is blocked. The face is hot, flushed, dark red and looks like that of fool. The skin is very hot. The temperature goes up. There is itching and tickling in the soft palate, in the throat and in the nasopharynx. The throat feels rough; it burns. At times there is the feeling of a lump in the throat, which cannot be swallowed. There is pain in the temples, in the throat, radiating towards the ear. The entire system of the ears, nose and throat appears to be affected.

Gelsemium acts as a prophylactic against flu.

The cold begins with dullness, a feeling of drowsiness, and sometimes even trembling. It comes on with degree of slowness. Complaints of Gelsemium are congestive complaints manifested through the brain and the spinal cord. The patient complains of a feeling of congestion as if somebody is tightening a band around his head. The eyes may be engorged and the pupils dilated. The eyes burn and itch. There is a chill running up the back from the lower part of the spine to the base of the head. There is trembling as if somebody was rubbing ice up the back. There may be various degrees of motor paralysis of the muscles about the eye, the throat, the chest, the larynx, the sphincter or the urethra. The patient suffers from muscular weakness and loss of muscular co-ordination. " Muscles will not obey the will". Gelsemium relieves 'writers' cramp' in the muscles of the forearm.

In case fever has come, the patient feels relieved if held because he is trembling. There may be heat and sweat stages which would be long and exhausting. His chill is without thirst. It begins between the scapulae. It runs in waves from sacrum to occiput. When problems come which require Gelsemium, the eyelids feel heavy; the patient even keep them open. The fingers are not manageable. If the patient attempts to walk, the legs tremble. If he wants to produce the tongue, the tongue trembles.

Muscular soreness of the neck and the shoulders with pain in the occiput requires Gelsemium. (We may think of Rhus Tox or Eupatorium Perf in case the pain is excruciating.)

Gelsemium is pre - eminently a nerve remedy. It relieves neuralgia in various parts. The pain may be a dull aching all over; it may be a sudden and darting, so acute as to startle a person. There may be spasms or convulsions. Through all this, there would be a characteristic prostration or weakness.

Congestive headache where there is pain at the base of the brain requires Gelsemium. So does not vertigo, spreading from the occiput. The headache is dull and there is a feeling of being tired. At times, however, there is violent pain in the occiput. Every pulsation is felt like the blow of a hammer at the base of the skull. The patient feels better if he lies with his head raise upon a high pillow. He does not want to move. Even thinking aggravates his problem. The headache is relieved if the patient is able to pass urine freely.

In the eyes, there is orbital neuralgia with contraction and twitching of the muscles. Detached retina requires Gelsemium. Corrects blurring and discomfort in eyes. Deep inflammations, with haziness of the vitreous. Dim sighted; pupils dilated and insensible to light. Eyelids heavy patient can hardly open them.

In males if there is discharge without erection, Gelsemium helps. Spermatorrhoea without erections. Genitals cold and relaxed. Gonorrhoea first stage; discharge scanty; little pain but much heat, smarting at meatus.

In women Gelsemium relieves false labour pains. It helps relax the painful spasm in the vagina known as vaginismus. Dsymenorrhoea, with scanty flow; menses retarded. Sensation as if uterus were squeezed.

Patient feels as if it was necessary to keep in motion, or else heart's action would cease. Slow pulse. Palpitation; pulse soft, weak full and flowing. Pulse slowly when quiet, but greatly accelerated on motion. Weak, slow pulse of old age.

The patient is generally thirstless.

Recommended potency: 200

The patient is better: Bending forward, Passing copious urine, in open air, by continuous motion, Using stimulants.

The patient is worse: In damp weather, in the morning hours, Due to emotional shock, before a thunderstorm.

□□□

CHAPTER 67

Graphites

Like all the carbons, this remedy is an antipsoric of great power, but especially active in patients who are rather stout, of fair complexion, with tendency to skin affections and constipations, fat, chilly, and costive, with delayed menstrual history, take cold easily.

Children impudent, teasing, laugh at reprimands. Anaemia with redness of face. Tendency to obesity.

By and large, Graphites is a skin remedy. Eruptions oozing out at thick honey - like fluid require Graphites. Such eruptions may be on any part of the body. These would be especially found on or beyond the ears, on the head, the face and the genitals or on the eyelids.

Graphites is indicated in eczema of the legs where there is a thick oozing of sticky fluid. Eczema of the eyelids, where the eruptions are moist and the margins of the eyelids are fissured, also requires Graphites.

In eczema around the anus, in anal fissures with oozing, Graphites is a very useful remedy.

Dryness of inner ear. Cracking in ears when eating. Moisture and eruptions behind the ear. Hears well in noise. Hardness of hearing. Hissing in the ears. Thin, white, scaly membrane covering membrane tympani, like exfoliated epithelium. Fissures in and behind the ears.

Aversion to meat. Hot drinks disagree. Nausea and vomiting after each meal. Morning sickness during menstruation. Pressure in stomach. Burning in stomach, causing hunger. Eructation difficult. Constrictive pain in stomach. Stomach pain is temporarily relieved by eating, hot drinks especially milk and lying down. Pain of gas opposite the side on which he lies. Chronic diarrhoea, stools brownish, liquid, undigested and offensive.

In constipation where the stool is knotty and large, Graphites is indicated. Mucus threads unite the lumps in the stool at times. The passing of the stool is followed by pain.

Graphites is of great help in cracks in the female nipples, cracks around the mouth, between the toes, in the ends of the fingers and on the labia. In the fissures, which respond to Graphite, the pain is burning. The skin is sore. There is a feeling of stitching and tearing. But more than anything else, there is numbness.

On the skin where every little injury suppurates and ulcers discharge a glutinous fluid, Graphites is indicated. The ulcers are scabby and crusty.

There is a marked offensive smell in oozing in cases, which require the use of Graphites. This offensive odor can be from the ears, in nasal discharge, the menstrual flow, ulcers and even in perspiration.

An excellent use of Graphites has been found in the treatment of fingernails and toenails which become thick and grow out of shape.

Graphites is useful in recurrent herpes upon any part of the body, but especially about the anus and the genitals. From the anus, there is a copious discharge of very offensive wind all the time Graphites help.

Mentally the patient is depressed. He thinks only of death and salvation. Unable to decide. Music makes her weep.

Pain in nape of neck, shoulders and back and limbs. Pain in small of back with great weakness. Left hand numb, arms feel sleep. Odema of lower limbs. Stiffness and contraction of toes. Cracks and fissures in ends of fingers.

Rush of blood to head with flushed face also with nosebleed and distension and flatulence. Headache in morning on wakening, especially on one side, with inclination to vomit. Rheumatic pains on one side of head, extending to teeth and neck. Burning on vertex. Humid, inching eruption on hairy scalp, emitting a fetid odor.

Menses too late, with constipation; pale and scanty with tearing pain in epigastria. Itching in vagina before menses. Hoarseness, coryza, cough, sweats and morning sickness during menstruation. Leucorrhoea, pale, thin, profuse, white, excoriating with great weakness in back. Mammae swollen and hard. In duration of ovaries and uterus and mammae. Nipples sore, cracked and blistered. Aversion to coitus.

Sexual weakness, with increased desire; aversion to coition; too early or no ejaculation. Herpetic eruption on organs.

Constriction of chest; spasmodic asthma, suffocative attacks wake from sleep; must eat something. Pain in middle of chest, with cough, scraping and soreness. Chronic hoarseness with skin affections. Hoarseness on beginning to sing. Cannot tolerate followers. Nose sore on blowing; is painful internally.

Graphites cures complaints of many kinds when two things are present:

1st The peculiar tendency to obesity.

2nd The characteristic glutinous eruptions.

Eczema of lids, eruptions moist and fissures red margins of lids covered with scales and crusts. In sulphur the margins are very red. All the orifices under sulphur are very red. Graphites lead all the remedies for eczematous affections of the lids.

Graphites is a deep acting, chronic remedy.

Recommended potency : 200, 1000. In case of sore nipples, apply mother tincture dissolved in water.

The patient is better: In warm clothing, in the dark and waking up.

The patient is worse from cold in winter, from heat in summer, in a warm room, in a warm bed and morning and evening.

□□□

CHAPTER 68

Hepar Sulphuris

Suits especially scrofulous and lymphatic constitutions that are inclined to have eruptions and glandular swellings. Unhealthy skin. Blondes with sluggish character and weak muscles. Great sensitiveness to all impressions. Sweating patient pulling blanket around him. Chilliness, hypersensitiveness, splinter-like pains, craving for sour and strong things are very characteristic. The tendency to suppuration is more marked, and ahs been a strong guiding symptom in practice. The side of the body on which he lies at night becomes gradually insufferably painful; he must turn.

Hepar Sulph is the medicine for abscess, for the tendency to suppuration. Every little injury suppurates. Accompanying this suppuration is shooting pain. Suppuration or pus formation can be on any part of the body. If throbbing and shooting pain accompany it, it requires a does of Hepar Sulph in a high potency of 200 and above. Hepar Sulph can abort pus formation if given at the earliest stage of suppuration. Later it will hasten the pointing and discharge and help in healing the ulcer.

The pain in which Hepar Sulph is indicated is very severe, very sharp. Whether there is an eruption or a boil, when pus has been formed, the pain is so intense that it is unbearable. It feels as if a sharp stick is piercing the skin.

A very important feature of situations where Hepar Sulph is a remedy is that the patient is chilly, is sensitive to cold and wants an unusual amount of clothing when in cold air. His sleeping room should be warm. He can tolerate a lot more heat than a person who is healthy and normal.

Sensitivity to impressions is a characteristic of a Hepar Sulph case. The patient is hypersensitive to touch, to pain, to cold air. Even if the pain is slight, the patient feels it and faints. On the inflamed parts even a touch of the hand is not bearable.

Unhealthy skin requires Hepar Sulph. The skin is chapped, with deep cracks on the hands and the feet. Ulcers on the skin, which bleeds with shooting, piercing pain, require Hepar Sulph.

Hepar Sulph is needed for chronic and recurring urticaria.

In persons where there is a constant offensive exhalation from the body, profuse sweat that is sour and offensive, Hepar Sulph is indicated. Patients who sweat day and night without relief are greatly helped by Hepar Sulph.

In Hepar, the skin is unhealthy, suppurating, moist and intensely sensitive to touch. In Sulphur, the skin eruptions are dry, itching and not sensitive to touch.

Hepar Sulph can take out foreign bodies known or unknown under the skin. In this it compares well with Silicea. That remedy is also capable of creating inflammation and suppuration in order to remove little foreign bodies that cannot be easily located.

Hepar Sulph and Silicea are distinguished by the modality that a Hepar patient is better in dry, warm weather. He has general sweats night and day. A Silicea patient has profuse head sweats at night and his foot sweats are offensive. Gland suppurations of Silicea are slow while those of Hepar are sudden and rapid. A Silicea patient wants self-confidence. The Hepar patient is sensitive beyond all bounds of reason. In the treatment of suppuration, Hepar Sulph comes at a stage earlier than that of Silicea.

Hepar Sulph helps in cases where the patients nose get stuffed every time he goes out in the cold air. There is a smell like that of old cheese. Hepar Sulph 1 X will often start secretion and profuse drainage in stuffy cold. Soreness of nostrils, with catarrhal troubles. Nose stopped up every time he goes out into cold air.

The discharge of foul-smelling pus from the ears responds to Hepar Sulph. Pustules in the auditory canals require Hepar Sulph. In the middle ear, an abscess may form. The ear drums ruptures. There may be bloody discharge with sticking, tearing pain in the inflamed ears.

When the throat is extremely sensitive to touch, it pains as if splinters are piercing the skin, and there is pus formation, Hepar Sulph is necessary. It is a must in quinsy unless the throat is purple whereupon Lachesis is needed. It is needed in chronic hypertrophy of the tonsils. Dry hoarse cough. Cough excited whenever any part of the body gets cold or uncovered, or from eating anything cold. Asthma worse in dry cold air; better in damp. Palpitation of heart. Hoarseness, with loss of voice. Rattling, croaking coughs; suffocative attacks have to rise up and bend head backwards.

In swollen glands with shooting, splinter pain Hepar Sulph is almost the only remedy available. The suppuration and pain can be in the glands of the neck, the axilla, the groin or of the female breast. First there is hard swelling with a feeling of sticks piercing it. Then comes a high inflammation and redness over the parts. Ultimately, there is suppuration and a consequent discharge. It may happen even in bones, around the roots of the nails and the ends of the fingers. He par Sulph is a great remedy in all such circumstances.

For women, Hepar Sulph helps abscess of the labia with great sensitivity. Leucorrhoea, which is offensive and smells like old cheese, also requires Hepar Sulph.

We have stated above that the Hepar Sulph patient is aggravated by cold air. This is so of the Aconite patient also. But in Hepar Sulph cases, the aggravation from cold air comes in the early morning hours while in Aconite it happens in the evenings and after sleep.

Herpes, sensitive, bleed easily. Ulcers externally on prepuce similar to chancre. Itching of glans, fraenum and scrotum. Suppurating inguinal glands. Humid soreness on genitals and between scrotum and thigh. Obstinate gonorrhoea "does not get well".

Micturition impeded. Patient is obliged to wait a while before the urine passes, and then it flows slowly for many days. Weakness of the bladder, the urine drops vertically down. Patient is never able to finish urinating; it seems as if some urine always remain behind in the bladder.

Recommended potency : 200 and higher.

The patient is better in damp weather, by wrapping his head up, from warmth and after eating.

The patient is worse from dry cold winds, from the least draught, touch, lying on painful side and early morning hours.

□□□

CHAPTER 69

Ipecacuanha

The name Ipecacuanha is from the Portuguese meaning, 'Road-side-sick-making plant', and mention of it as a remedy for the bloody flux or dysentery goes back as far as the late sixteenth century.

The principle feature of Ipecacuahna is its persistent nausea and vomiting, which form the chief guiding symptom. Indicated after indigestible food, raisins, cakes, etc. especially indicated in fat children and adults, who are feeble and catch cold in relaxing atmosphere, warm moist weather.

One cannot think of treating persistent nausea without Ipecac. This is a nausea in which there is no relief by vomiting. The patient is as sick after as before. The second major problem for which Ipecac is a great cure is a chest complaint, bronchitis in infants, bronchitis with coarse rattling. Ipecac is also a remedy for infections of the upper respiratory tract wherein a peculiar wheezing sound is produced on breathing out. Old incurable cases of asthma are relieved by Ipecac. Ipecac is useful in uterine haemorrhages.

A patient who suffers from nausea in any sickness, whether or not connected with the gastric system, requires a dose of Ipecac.

Women vomit during pregnancy. At that time, think of Ipecac.

Unyielding cases of gastritis where even a drop of water will not stay down. The patient vomits everything that he takes. There is a sharp pain in the stomach, going from left to right, and pain in the back. The vomit consists of bile. The nausea is without a pause.

Like Pulsatilla, Ipecac is indicated after taking indigestible food like raisins, cakes and fats. For children particularly, Ipecac can avoid the development of the trouble into an obstinate gastroenteritis or cholera infantum, if a dose in 200 potency is given. There is colic pain, cutting pain, going from left to right. In such cases, the stool is characteristic. It is fermented, foamy like yeast; there is mucus. The colour is grass green and sometimes blood is present. In Pulsatilla cases, the tongue are often coated, while in Ipecac cases, the tongue is, by and large, perfectly clean.

In gastric disturbances, as Dr. E.B. Nash has put it, Pulsatilla may be considered a better choice while the food is in the stomach and is not being thrown out. Ipecac would be the choice when even after the food is out, the nausea persists.

The Ipecac affections of the respiratory organs also are accompanied by nausea. During nausea, the face turns pale, the eyes sunken, with blue margins. A violent degree of dsypnoea, of difficulty in breathing with wheezing and a great weight on the chest accompanies bronchitis.

For wheezing, the first medicine to be thought of is Ipecac. (If there is coarse rattling and there is accumulation of mucus in the chest, the indicated medicine is Antim Tart 200, 1000).

Ipecac is invaluable in respiratory problems where there is a constant constriction in the chest. The patient suffers from asthma. There is incessant cough, which is violent. He has to cough with every breath. Before the mucus has been formed, Ipecac gives tremendous relief. Later, when the chest appears to be full of phlegm, which does not come out on coughing, Ipecac still helps. There may be a complete loss of voice called 'aphonia'. At times, there is bleeding from lungs with nausea besides the feeling of constriction. An asthma patient should always have Ipecac 30 and Aconite 30 with him. The two medicines cab be alternated when the attack comes, and continued at 15 minutes interval till the patient obtains relief.

As stated above, Ipecac is a great friend of the infant. In infantile pneumonia where the chest is loaded with mucus, where there is rapid, wheezing respiration, where the face is turning blue or pale, Ipecac should be instantly administered.

In infants, bad colds end in chest troubles, which are characterized as bronchitis. There is cough, with pain below the ribs. There is a coarse rattling, which can be heard throughout the room. The trouble comes on pretty rapidly. The child looks pale and sick. Ipecac gives him comfort. If there is too much of rattling, Antimonium Tart symptoms come on slowly. That is the difference, besides the extent of rattling, in the use of these two medicines.

For whooping cough, administer Ipecac when there is nausea, violent whooping, convulsions, thirstlessness, spasms, a red face and vomiting of all food taken in.

Active, profuse, bright red haemorrahage from any orifice of the body responds well to Ipecac. Nausea and heavy breathing can from the nose, the lungs, the stomach, the womb, the kidneys, the bladder or the rectum, ever accompany the haemorrahage.

When there is a sudden uterine haemorrhage, gushing blood flowing in large quantities, invariably accompanied by nausea, Ipecac is the remedy. There is a pain from the navel to the uterus. The blood is bright red.

Ipecac is of great use in amoebic dysentery with tenesmus. When the patient strains to let the stool out, he feels nauseated. The pain is cutting. It is worse around the navel. The patient is almost constantly on the commode but passes a little slime, a little blood each time.

Headache with nausea is relieved by Ipecac. The pain in the skull - bone is crushing and extends to the teeth and to the root of the tongue.

Fever; particularly intermittent fever, which comes with periodicity, when it is accompanied by nausea, is relieved by Ipecac. In a typical Ipecac fever there are chill as well as heat, nausea, vomiting and breathlessness.

In Ipecac cases thirstlessness is common.

Recommended potency: 200,1000.

The patient is worse: In moist, warm weather, lying down, intermittently.

CHAPTER 70

Kali Bichromicum

Kali Bi is one of the finest remedies for the treatment of sinusitis, in diphtheric croup and in chronic, old cases. The mucous membrane of the nose responds to the administration of Kali Bi in acute as well as chronic cases. The discharge is tough, stringy, green and goes inwards into the throat.

The mucus is very difficult to take out. The patient can be heard from a distance trying to take it out but without success. One dose of Kali Bi. loosens this mucus.

There is pain in the sinuses. There is neuralgia in the orbits above the eyes. The sense of smell has been lost. The nose is stuffed. At times, there is violent sneezing. The patient suffers from chronic inflammation of the frontal sinuses. Only Kali Bi. gives relief and cure to such a patient.

Catarrhal laryngitis cough has a brassy sound. True membranous croup, extending to larynx and nares. Cough with pain in sternum, extending to shoulders. Pain at bifurcation of trachea on coughing from midsternum to back.

Some other symptoms are also there in cases of the type indicated above. There is headache above the eyebrows. In the frontal bone, above the nose and between the eyes, there is continuous, aching pain. More so on the right side. The bones and the scalp feel sore. Snuffles of children, especially fat, chubby babies. Fetid smell. Discharge thick, ropy, greenish yellow. Tough, elastic plugs from nose; leave a raw surface. Inability to breathe through nose. Coryza, with obstruction of nose. Violent sneezing. Profuse, watery nasal discharge. Chronic inflammation of frontal sinus with stopped up sensation.

When the eyes discharge ropy and yellow mucus, when the ears are swollen, have sharp stitching pain, often with thick, yellow and stingy discharge, and Kali Bi comes into help. In a descending aircraft excruciating pain comes in the ears. This requires a dose of Kali Bi. half - an -hour before descent. Its use over a few days eliminates this discomfort because the sinuses are cleared of the tough mucus.

Tonsils are inflamed, swollen, and red. The uvula is bloated like a balloon but relaxed. There is intense pain at the root of the tongue. Tough, ropy, mucus flows down the throat. Use Kali BI. fauces red and inflamed. Parotids glands swollen.

Kali Bi cures thick, ropy and green discharges from the nose, the mouth, the fauces, the pharynx, and the larynx. The trachea, the bronchia, the vagina and the uterus. From any mucus membrane.

Kali Bi cures ulceration of the mucous membranes. These ulcers form as a consequence of the ropy, green discharge, have regular edges, as if cut with a punch. At times, tough membranes from Kali Bi take care of them.

In chronic cold with the other symptoms indicated above, there might be formation of tough, green, hard plugs in the nose. Simultaneously, there is a flow of thick, ropy mucus into the throat. Kali Bi is indicated.

Similarly, diphtheric membranes formed in the throat and extending downwards into the larynx respond very well to Kali Bi.

When headache is preceded by blindness, Kali Bi. has been found to be an effective remedy. The blindness disappears after the headache begins. The pain settles in a small spot and is intense.

Think of Kali Bi in perforation of the septum.

Kali bi is also of great help in the following conditions:

Chronic intestinal ulceration with cutting pain in the abdomen soon after eating.

Ropy mucus in urine. After urinating, a drop seems to remain which cannot be expelled. There is pain in the coccyx before urinating, with relief thereafter. Congestion of kidneys; nephritis, with scanty, albuminous urine and casts. Pyelitis, urine mixed with epithelial cells, mucus, pus or blood.

A yellow, ropy and tenacious leucorrhoea, with intense itching of the vulva.

Left sided severe sciatica. Better by motion. Worse during hot weather. Tearing pain in tibia. Wandering rheumatic pain in joints with swelling, heat and redness. Cracking in joints. Bones feel sore and bruised. Pain, swelling and stiffness and crackling of all joints. Pains fly rapidly from one place to another. Wandering pains along the bones; worse from cold.

Tendo-Achillies; tendon is swollen and painful. Soreness of heels with weakness. Pain along the bones is worse on exposure.

Eczema of the scalp, with thick, heavy crusts oozing a thick, glutinous substance. Acne. Ulcer with punched out edges, with tendency to penetrate and tenacious exudation. Itching with vesicular eruption.

Like Belladonna the Kali Bichromium pain appears and disappears suddenly. Like Pulsatilla, this pain flits from place to place in the body. However, in Pulsatilla the green mucus is bland and comes out easily in direct contrast to Kali Bi mucus, which is difficult to take out.

Recommended potency: 200. Higher in severe sinus pain.

The patient is better from heat.

The patient is worse in the morning, in hot weather, while undressing, catches cold quickly and is sensitive to cold.

CHAPTER 71

Lachesis

Like all snake poisons, Lachesis decomposes the blood rendering it more fluid; hence a haemorrhagic tendency is marked. Purpura, septic states, diphtheria, and other low forms of disease when the system is thoroughly poisoned and the prostration is marked. Delirium tremens with much trembling and confusion. Very important medicine during menopause and for patients of a melancholic disposition. Diphtheria carriers. Sensation of tension in various parts.

Lachesis treats the worst of throat problems, hot flushes in women during menopause, and diptheric paralysis. It is indicated in high blood pressure with constriction and in heart disease when the face is purple and bloated. Also religious insanity.

As a red inflammation leads us to use Belladonna, so Lachesis is to be thought of when the colour is purple. The face is purple; the eyes are engorged. An inflamed spot is purple and so are the inflamed glands. Ulceration bleeds, blood coagulates and the surface looks purple. There is extreme sensitivity to touch. The throat is purple and not red because the blood under the skin has coagulated. There is nothing like Lachesis if these indications are present.

'Constriction is present in most problems where Lachesis is indicated.

Lachesis is a snake poison and in pure form decomposes the blood, making its flow easy. In haemorrhage, it cures such circumstances. Persistent bleeding easily started. Cancers turn bluish black, bleed copiously, frequently and burn.

A Lachesis patient suffers an aggravation in the spring when he goes from cold weather into milder weather. He is worse at the end of sleep or on taking a warm bath. He is afraid to go to sleep because his condition worsens.

A Lachesis patient suffers from insanity in which religious feelings overwhelm. He is loquacious. He believes that he is in supreme human control and obeying commands. He thinks that he has a hot-line to GOD. Such a patient is full of conceit, envy, hatred, revenge and cruelty.

Another may be ecstatic, prophetic and be in a trance.

Still others have jealousy without basis. An unnecessary apprehension of the future.

Lachesis is needed to cure a mania to go on talking, sense or nonsense. Volubility with a puzzling lack of sequence.

As mentioned above, Lachesis has an excellent effect in throat problems. The pain starts left, runs from throat into the ears. The patient feels so choked that he wants to loosen his collar. Quinsy has set in. there is difficulty in swallowing liquids. Hot drinks are uncomfortable. The throat is painful to the touch. Swallowing saliva or liquids aggravates the pain more than the swallowing of solids. The throat looks purple.

Lachesis takes care of a tendency to chronic sore throat and ulceration. Red and grey ulceration; deep ulceration; with patches full of pus. It is a medicine for diphtheria, which commences on the left side and spreads to the right. The membrane is dusky, blackish. The inflammations of the tonsils also spread in a similar fashion. At the same time the pharynx might be full of thick, white, ropy mucus in the morning. Paralysis of the vocal cods, when the voice is lost, needs Lachesis. The larynx is sensitive to the slightest touch. It is constricted.

Any disease, which spends its main force in the throat, whether pneumonia or typhoid, responds to Lachesis.

In heart problems, acute or chronic, the patient suffers an attack of suffocation. His cough comes with pain in the anus or with stitches in the piles if he has them. He feels constriction. His blood pressure is high. There is a rush of blood to the head. The patient has palpitation. His feet are cold.

Similarly in an attack of asthma, where there is a sudden flush of heat, orgasm of blood, threatened paralysis of lungs or heart, where the patient wants to loosen clothes to prevent suffocation, Lachesis should be thought of.

Desperate cases of croup where the child gets worse in sleep are cured by administration of Lachesis.

Menopause in women is seldom trouble free. They suffer from flushes of heat, uterine haemorrahge, palpitation, fainting spells and suffocation in warm rooms. These women experience pressure on the vertex; even burning. The patient dislikes the pressure of clothes. She has haemorrhoids. Lachesis is a sure remedy.

Purple inflammation, may be cancerous, of the mammae is relieved by Lachesis. So is inflammation of the left ovary where the ovary is swollen, painful and hard. Cancer of the left ovary spreading to the right from left needs Lachesis.

Lachesis relieves varicose veins during pregnancy. Blue or purple, very sensitive to touch, but relieved by pressure.

Sunstroke: Lachesis is a great remedy for headache, which comes after a person, has moved in the sun. But to relieve the immediate effect of sunstroke, Glonoine is the first remedy. If a person gets headache on the least exposure to the sun's heat, use Lachesis as a chronic cure.

Lachesis relieves trifacial neuralgia on the left side with heat running up into the head. There is tearing pain in the jaw-bones. The face is purple, swollen and looks jaundiced.

Lachesis relieves neuralgic pain in the coccyx if the pain is worse on rising from a sitting posture and better on sitting perfectly still.

Paralysis of the left side of the body, later extending to the right side responds well to the use of Lachesis.

In gum-problems, Lachesis follows Merc. Sol very well. The gums are swollen, spongy and bleed easily. When the gums turn purple. Lachesis to be used.

Lachesis is a remarkably effective remedy for erysipelas, for malignant boils and gangrenous affections. The affected parts have a purple appearance. The patient is sensitive to touch. There is swelling, bluish turning into black.

Recommended Potency 200 and higher.

The patient is better: Loosening clothes, by onset of discharge, for instance, menses nasal flow, warm application.

The patient is worse: In spring, at the end of sleep.

CHAPTER 72

Lycopodium Clavatum

The word LYCOPODIUM is derived from LUCOS meaning wolf and PES meaning the foot, as the shoots has an appearance of the wolf's foot. CLAVATUM derived from Latin word CLAVATUS meaning club-like.

This drug is inert until the spores are crushed. Its wonderful medicinal properties are only disclosed by trituration and succussion. In nearly all cases where Lycopodium is the remedy, some evidence of urinary or digestive disturbance will be found. Lycopodium is adapted more especially to ailments gradually developing functional powers, where the function of the liver is seriously disturbed. Atony. Malnutrition. Mild temperaments of lymphatic constitution, with catarrhal tendencies; older persons, where the skin shows yellowish spots, earthy complexion, uric acid diathesis, etc.; also precocious, weak children. Symptoms characteristically run from right to left, act especially on right side of body, and are worse from 4 to 8 PM.

Lycopodium is most useful in troubles relating to digestion. These troubles arise from the consumption of food, which ferments in the digestive system. That is why Lycopodium relieves a bloated and full abdomen wherein the wind is pressing downwards.

It may not be out of place to mention here that Carbo Veg. Overall flatulence is relieved by China relieves flatulence pressing upwards. Flatulence pressing downwards is relieved by Lycopodium.

When even a small intake of food creates a feeling of flatulence, Lycopodium is indicated. Food tastes sour in such cases and there are burning eructation.

When the patient experiences incessant fermentation of food in the abdomen, as if yeast is in action, we should think of Lycopodium.

Dr. J.T. Kent has described the flatulence of the Lycopodium patient in the following words: "Distended like a drum so that he can hardly breathe. The diaphragm pushed upwards, infringing upon the lungs and heart space so that he has palpitation, faintness and dyspnoea." Everything that such a person takes turns into wind. The pressure is downwards.

Patients of chronic liver trouble suffer from flatulence quite often. They have pain shooting across the lower abdomen from right to leave. The liver is sensitive. At times, there is dropsy due to a sluggish liver. There are brown spots on the abdomen. Lycopodium is the medicine in such cases.

For chronic appendicitis, use Lycopodium. Pain shoots across the lower abdomen from right to leave.

Similarly, Lycopodium helps in cases of haemorrhoids, which are very painful to touch and which are found in patients with chronic liver trouble and flatulence.

In cases of constipation, Lycopodium helps if for days the patient has had no desire to pass stool. His insides are full but there is no urge. When the stool passes, the first part is hard but the later part is soft and gushing.

Lycopodium has been found to be greatly effective in the cure of impotency. Dr. E.B.Nash puts it thus in his inimitable style: "An old man marries his second or third wife and finds himself not equal to the occasion. It is very embarrassing for the whole family. A dose of Lycopodium sets the thing right and makes the doctor a warm friend on both sides of the house." One dose of 10,000 potency once a week is advisable.

In women, Lycopodium is a remedy when the vagina is dry and on that account, sexual intercourse is painful. Not only that, there is burning in the vagina during and after coition.

Varicose veins of pudenda respond well to Lycopodium.

Lycopodium is the medicine for eczematous eruptions behind the ears, on smooth hairless patches on the skull and on the face. The eruptions on the face are of copper colour. In these cases eczema is associated with urinary, gastric and liver problems.

Lycopodium helps when the patient is melancholy, apprehensive, is confused, and has lost self-confidence. His brainpower is failing. He is irritable and peevish; he cannot endure opposition.

In old people when the memory fails, when an old person uses wrong words, spells wrongly and is unable to do ordinary mental work, Lycopodium is useful.

Lycopodium should not be forgotten in chronic dry catarrh of the nose. At night, particularly, the patient has to breathe through the mouth because the nose is completely blocked.

In infants, the chest is full of mucus and rattling noises are heard. The child wheezes while breathing out. Lycopodium helps.

Recommended potency: 200. But in not -too- frequent doses.

The patient is better: After midnight, in motion, in cool, open air, from being uncovered, In throat and abdomen by warm drinks.

The patient is worse : In the afternoon, 4.00 to 8.00 PM, After eating, In a warm room, heat, hot air, in bed, From right to left, from above downwards, From warm applications except throat and abdomen.

❑❑❑

CHAPTER 73

Mercurius Solubilis

Every organ and tissue of the body is more or less affected by this powerful drug; it transforms healthy cells into inflamed and necrotic cells; decomposes the blood producing a profound anaemia. This is converted into useful life saving and life preserving service if employed homoeopathically, guided by its clear-cut symptoms. The lymphatic system is especially affected with all the membranes and glands, and internal organs, bones, etc. lesions produced by Mercury are very similar to those of syphilis. Very often indicated in the secondary stage of syphilis where there is a febrile chloroanaemia, rheumatoid pains around joints, etc. all mercury symptoms are worse at night, from warmth of bed, from damp, cold, rainy weather, worse during perspiration. It is also known as human 'thermometre'. Sensitive to heat and cold. Breath, excretions and body smell foul. Tendency to pus formation, which is thin, greenish, putrid, streaked with thin blood.

We think of Merc Sol in mucous dysentery, pus formation anywhere, particularly in the tonsils, gum problems, painful ulcers in the mouth and in a very uncomfortable running nose. A tendency to ulcerate, or to formation of pus, requires Merc Sol.

Mercury is sensitive to temperature, to heat and to cold. So is the mercurius patient. He is worse from extremes of both heat and cold. A warm room and a warm bed aggravate the problem and naturally these troubles are worse at night. The patient perspires profusely without relief. He experiences a creeping chilliness in fever. His skin is almost all the time moist because of day and night sweating. Persistent sweating without relief in any problem indicates Merc Sol.

In problems, which can be dealt with by Merc Sol, an offensive odour rises all through whether; it is in the urine or the stool or in the sweat. Nasal as well as mouth diseases have a fetid odour.

A remarkable cure of Merc Sol is of the tendency to the formation of pus. The pus is thin, green, and foul smelling and sometimes streaked with thin blood. The abscesses burn and sting. (In case the pus has a shooting pain, the use of Hepar Sulph is advisable). Inflammations of joints, of cavities of the pleura have this pus.

Merc Sol does wonders in ulcers in the mouth, painful ulcers, where there is foul breath. There are blisters filled with pus or wounds, which are painful. These ulcers can be on the gums, on the lips and the inside of the cheeks. The tongue is ulcerated and swollen. The teeth leave an imprint on the tongue. Fetid saliva needs Merc. Sol. a foul odour from the mouth that can be smelt all over the room. In Merc. A Sol case there is a great thirst for cold drinks even when the mouth is moist.

Swollen, itching, spongy and bleeding gums have their cure in Merc Sol. The teeth are loose, black or dirty. The gums are painful to touch. A sensation of severe itching or pulsation is felt in the gums and the roots. The gums have a blue-red margin or are purple in colour. Abscesses of the gums and of the roots of the teeth find a cure in Merc- Sol.

In tonsils where pus has formed, but as yet there is no shooting pain, Merc Sol immediately gives relief. There may be fever with gripping chilliness and sweat. The condition of the patient is worse in the evening and worsens into the night. (If it were a shooting, digging pain, Hepar Sulph would be the remedy.)

The tonsils are swollen, red with pale patches. If the tonsils in the throat turn purple, Lachesis would be the medicine.) After pus has formed, swallowing is difficult, painful. At times, there is a complete loss of voice.

For mucous dysentery, Merc Sol is the first medicine to be thought of. The stool is slimy, at times bloody. There is tenesmus that is a feeling of 'cannot finish' though not so severe and intolerable as in Merc Cor. This dysentery causes cutting colic in the abdomen, a rumbling distension, aches and pain.

In ear troubles, where there is a foul smelling discharge of green, thick and corrosive pus from the ears, Merc Sol is a cure. So, too, in otitis media with ruptured drum. The ear infection causes stinging pain. In an overall view the remedy here is Merc Sol and not Apis.

Merc Sol cures a thick, green, yellow, corrosive and foul smelling discharge from the nose. The nasal bones have been affected. There might be even a bloody discharge from the nose. Non-stop thin running nose responds to Merc-Sol.

Cold spreads from the nose to the eye in patients suffering from gout and rheumatic pain. Purulent opthalamia with swollen lids needs Merc Sol. In such cases, Merc Sol cures iritis. It is also indicated for inflammation of the cornea.

Inflammatory rheumatism with much swelling, aggravated by the heat of the bed and from uncovering responds well to Merc Sol.

Glandular inflammation with hardness requires Merc. Sol. Inflammation of the mammae, the parotids (near the ear), sublingual (beneath the tongue), lymphatic glands of the neck, groin and axilla, even the liver. Skin inflammations when hard need this remedy.

Merc. Sol is a palliative in cancer of the mammae and of the uterus.

Intense thirst and hunger : The Merc. Sol patient has an intense thirst for cold drinks. He is always hungry.

Recommended potency : 200 and above.

Patient is better from cold drinks. Next time patient is worse in Wet, damp weather; in cold open air, at night, lying on the right side, in a warm room and in warm bed.

□□□

CHAPTER 74

Natrum Muriaticum

The prolong taking of excessive salt causes profound nutritive changes to take place in the system, and there arises not only the symptoms of salt retention as evidenced by dropsies and oedemas, but also an alteration in the blood causing a condition of anaemia and leucocytosis. There seems also to be retention in the tissues. It is a great remedy for certain forms of intermittent fever, anaemia, chlorosis, many disturbances of the alimentary tract and skin. Great debility; most weakness felt in the morning in bed. Dry mucous membranes. Constrictive sensation throughout the body. Great weariness and weakness. Oversensitive to all sorts of influences. Hyperthyroidism. Goiter, Addison's disease. Diabetes.

According to Dr. E.B. Nash, Nat Mur is one of the best homoeopathic remedies for anemia. This anaemia can be caused by loss of fluids, by menstrual irregularities, by grief or mental diseases. The patient is pale, emaciated and in spite of eating very well he is anaemic. He suffers from a throbbing headache, soreness while climbing steps, exhaustion or physical exertion, constipation to some degree and overall depression. Some women have scanty flow of blood during menses.

In cases of anaemia, which respond to Nat Mur there is always palpitation, great fluttering of the heart. It is an excellent remedy in tachycardia, that is, in cases of abnormally rapid heartbeat. Sensations of coldness of the heart and of constriction are present.

Another effective use of Nat Mur is in cases of violent and fluent running nose, coryza, which lasts from one to three days. Often, the nose gets stuffed making breathing difficult. Nat Mur is infallible for stopping a cold commencing with sneezing. There is loss of smell and taste. Discharge thin and watery, like raw white of an egg.

In unyielding cases of intermittent fever, Nat Mur in 200 and higher potencies is of great help. Chronic malarial states with weakness, constipation, and loss of appetite respond to Nat Mur. Around the mouth there could be pearl-like blisters.

Nat Mur is an excellent remedy for periodic chills. The chill can come everyday, every other day, every third or fourth day in the morning about 10. 30 a.m. the chill begins in the extremities which becomes blue. There is a throbbing headache. The patient is thirsty for cold water, although he is suffering from great chill; but there is no thirst during fever. His teeth chatter. He rolls from side to side. His bones ache. The fever is so high that the fingers are scorching. The fever is relieved by sweat and so is aching. You can call it malaria or any other fever. The medicine is Nat Mur.

In intermittent fevers a blinding headache where the pain is that of a hundred little hammers knocking on the head, responds very well to Nat Mur. The headache comes after menstruation, lasts sunrise to sunset. The same is true of chronic headache and congestive headache, which are present from sunrise to sunset. The patient would have simultaneously a pale face. He has nausea and even vomits. He is worse from noise, from music and from a warm room, worse even lying down. He feels better in the open air, from cold baths.

Eyes feel bruised with headache in school children. Eyelids heavy. Muscles weak and stiff. Letters run together. Burning in eyes. Lacrymation, burning and acrid. Lids swollen. Eyes appear wet with tears. Tears stream down face on coughing. Pain in eyes when looking down.

Mental depression on account of suffering in chronic diseases is an important in cases where Nat Mur is indicated. The patient's depression is aggravated by consolation. (In Pulsatilla consolation ameliorates.)

Nat Mur is useful in dropsy of the brain following meningeal diseases. In acute spinal meningitis, with chronic jerking of the head. It is useful in oedema of the lower extremities.

Nat Mur is indicated in numbness and tingling in the fingers and the lower extremities of the knees, legs, feet. The palms are hot and perspiring. The ankles are weak and turn easily. Numbness in the lips and the tongue also responds to Nat Mur. Backache relieved by firm support needs Nat Mur. Painful contraction of hamstrings.

Abnormal craving for salt is taken care of by Nat Mur, thus proving the principle of 'Like cures like.

Nat Mur helps in cases of constipation where there is an obstinate retention of stools. The rectum is in active. The anus is torn and bleeding. The stool may come out in large masses, but is difficult to expel.

Dryness of the mucous membranes anywhere in the body responds well to Nat Mur.

Skin is greasy, oily, especially on hairy parts. Dry eruptions, especially on margins of hairy scalp and bends of joints. Fever blisters. Urticaria itch and burn. Warts on palms of hand. Eczema; raw, red and inflamed. Alopecia.

Nat Mur is a long acting, deep acting remedy, which operates slowly and brings about its result after some time. But it does act in acute cases as well.

Recommended potency : 200 and higher.

The patient is better by pressure against aback, taking cold bath, in open air and by lying on right side.

The patient is worse about 10 a.m., by heat, in a warn room, form noise, from music, from talking, from mental exertion and from consolation.

❑❑❑

CHAPTER 75

Nitric Acid

The main action of this drug is on the outlets of the body where the mucous membrane and the skin meet; these pain as from splinters. Marked improvement of symptoms while riding in a carriage. Acts best on the dark complexioned and past middle life. Syphilis after abuse of mercury. Pains appear and disappear rapidly. All discharges very offensive especially urine, faeces, and perspiration. Persons who have chronic diseases and take cold easily and disposed to diarrhoea. Excessive physical irritability.

The human body has many outlets where the mucous membranes and the skin meet. Any pain on account of problems in these regions is severe. It is a sticking pain. It is a pain as if somebody is piercing the surface with splinters. Nitric Acid is the remedy for problems of this type.

The skin and the mucous membrane join at the corners of the mouth, in the nose and at the anus. On the lips the corners crack, get ulcerated and swollen. In the mouth there are blisters with a lot of pus and swelling. The gums are swollen, ulcerated and spongy. Fissures occur in the canthi. Nitric Acid is the first remedy in such cases.

Mentally, the patient requiring Nitric Acid is indifferent to all matters in life. He is tired of life. He is hopeless. Long suffering, pain and sickness have broken him. His suffering is more physical than mental. Anaemia and emaciation are marked. Patient is hopeless. Sensitive to noise, pain, touch and jar. Patient is irritable, hateful and vindictive.

This patient is sensitive to cold. He always feels chilly. All his symptoms are aggravated from loss of heat and in cool air. He is ever catching colds. No sooner does he get over one cold than he has another. There is coryza every winter. Nasal catarrh with offensive smell. Feeling of splinters in the nose. Obstructed, stuffed nose at night. Discharge yellow and offensive. Green crusts are blown out every morning. Administer Nitric Acid.

In the mouth if there are ulcers in the soft palate, with sharp splinter like pains, Nitric Acid is indicated.

In the throat when there are white patches with sharp pain, as from splinters, on swallowing, Nitric Acid gives relief.

Toothache which is tearing and which is aggravated from cold or warm things is relieved by Nitric Acid. The gums bleed easily. There is pulsation in the gums, in the evening and during the night. Nitric Acid helps in tooth decay. When Merc Sol Fails in toothache, use Nitric Acid.

Great hunger, with sweetish taste. Longing for indigestible things - chalk, earth etc. dyspepsia with excess of oxalic acid, uric acid and phosphates in urine and great mental depression. Loves fat and salt. Violent cutting pains after stools, lasting for hours. After stools, irritable and exhausted.

Nitric Acid is an excellent remedy in prolonged suppuration in glands with no tendency to repair, and when there are sticking pains.

For anal fissures, Nitric Acid is a medicine par excellence. There is severe pain after passage of stool, even soft stool.

Rectal problems have a special affinity for Nitric Acid. The patient suffers from a feeling of splinters in the rectum. After stool there is still an urging; there is exhaustion. There may be painful prolapse of the rectum. Nitric Acid is very effective in fistula, fissures, carbuncles, haemorrhages and even cancer of the rectum, when the symptoms of splinter pain, tenesmus, foul odour and an inability to heal early are present. The patient cries out if somebody touches the affected parts. The haemorrhoids are painful to touch. These bleed externally as well as internally, at the time of passing stool. The discharge of blood and pus is copious.

In cases requiring Ratanhia, there is a great constriction in the anus. There is burning like fire, temporarily relieved by cold water. The stool has to be forced with great effort. There are sudden knife - like stitches. The anus aches and burns for hours after stool. The rectum aches as if full of broken glass. Even in the stomach there is a pain like knives cutting deep. The cutting pain continues for hours after passing the stool under both the medicines. The burning feeling is absent in cases requiring Nitric Acid.

Nitric Acid is a very effective remedy when the odour in the urine is offensive. The urine itself is dark. It smells like horse urine. There is burning and sticking on urination.

Small ulcers on glans penis and on prepuce require Nitric Acid. A splinter-like sensation is present. Pimples, ulcers, herpes and crusts on the prepuce require Nitric Acid. The penis is in a constant state of irritability.

A feeling of splinters in the nipples of a woman, when the nipples are fissured and tender, would respond very favourably to Nitric Acid.

Nitric Acid discharges are offensive, weather of the urine, faeces or perspiration. The patient bleeds easily, profuse, dark blood. His eruptions foul smell difficult to heal.

Recommended potency: 30,200.

The patient is better: Riding in a carriage.

The patient is worse: In the evening, in the night, in cold climate, hot weather, from hot and cold drinks.

□□□

CHAPTER 76

Nux Vomica

The word NUX VOMICA is derived from Latin word NUX meaning nut and VOMERE meaning vomiting because of the peculiar property of the nut.

Is the greatest of polychrests, because the bulk of its symptoms correspond in similarity with those of the commonest and most frequent of diseases. It is frequently the first remedy, indicated after much dosing, establishing a sort of equilibrium of forces and counteracting chronic effects.

Nux is pre-eminently the remedy for many of the conditions incident to modern life. The typical Nux patient is thin, spare, quick, active, nervous and irritable. He does a good deal of mental work; has mental strains and leads a sedentary life, found in prolonged office work, over study and close application to business with cares and anxieties. This indoor life and mental strain seeks stimulants, coffee, wine, possibly in excess; or again, he hopes to quiet his excitement, by indulging in the sedative effects of tobacco, if not really a victim, to the seductive drugs, like opium etc. Nux is preeminently a male remedy. These conditions produce an irritable, nervous system, hypersensitive and over impressionable, which Nux will do much to soothe and calm. Especially adapted to digestive disturbances, portal congestion and hypochondriacal states depending thereon. Nux patients are easily chilled, avoid open air. Nux always seems to be out of tune, inharmonious spasmodic action.

In the entire homoeopathic materia medica if any medicine has been used more than others, it is Nux Vomica. Quite often, it is essential to administer this medicine first after a patient has been prescribed many other medicines in the other systems without having been cured. But more than anything else

Nux is a remedy par excellence for hangovers, dyspepsia, blind piles, colic and stuffy colds. It relieves gastric headaches.

Nux is the medicine for the modern man, the jet setter. He is fond of late nights, intoxicants normally leads a sedentary life and gets up with a hangover. He often keeps long office hours. In such a case, a does of Nux Vomica before going to bed would take care of the sleeplessness and of the morning hangover with a heavy head and indigestion.

The best remedy in such cases as mentioned above would of course, to modify one's habits. But in case troubles have arisen on account of the habits indicated above, Nux Vomica is the cure for the problems arising out of the use of the stimulants, the consumption of alcohol, narcotics, patent medicines, late nights, rich food and debauchery.

Mentally, the Nux Vomica patient is over-sensitive to a striking degree. He is easily irritated. He cannot bear noise. He is over-sensitive to medicines. Such a person does not like to be contradicted, scolds others unnecessarily.

Nux Vomica is an excellent cure in headache, which occurs along with gastric symptoms and with haemorrhoids. The headache increases from mental exertion, irritation, from fresh air or from the use of intoxicants and is there on waking up in the morning. Sun shine headaches respond well to Nux. So does vertigo after dinner or early morning on waking up. A momentary loss of consciousness may be experienced.

Nux Vomica has been noticed to have a remarkable effect on stuffy colds and snuffles caused by exposure to cold and dry atmosphere. The nose is bottled up at night and in fresh air. In children, the nose is blocked and dry. The child can hardly breathe. He breathes through his mouth. Nux gives quick relief.

The Nux patient sleeps by fits and starts and his sleep is such that he wakes up around 3.00AM and immediately all his problems converge on his thinking. This worrying wakefulness may continue till morning when fatigue might bring sleep. Nux Vomica is a sure cure in such cases. One dose at 3.00 a.m. or there about will recall soothing sleep.

The other important spheres of action of Nux Vomica are the stomach and abdomen. The patient has constipation. Although he has a frequent desire to pass stool, yet each time he passes only a small quantity of faeces.

For dysentery where Nux Vomica is a remedy, the pain is greatly relieved for only a short time after every motion.

Nux Vomica helps relieve colic pain in the abdomen. The pain is so cutting the patient feels forced to bend double.

Nux Vomica is an excellent remedy for blind haemorrhoids with itching, and an ineffectual urge to pass stool.

Backache, in the lumber region, often occurring in conjunction with piles is greatly helped by Nux Vomica.

A patient for whom Nux Vomica is indicated is generally worse in the morning, mentally as well as physically.

A patient with constant uneasiness in the rectum benefits greatly by the use of Nux Vomica. There is a feeling of pressure in the rectum all the time.

In menstrual disorders where the menses are always irregular, start too early, last too long, have black blood; Nux Vomica has been found to be extremely beneficial. In such cases, one menstrual cycle is virtually carried on into the next. An irascible, over sensitive to medicines, mental state would be a definite indication.

In menses, there may be pain in the sacrum and a constant urge to pass stool. With painful menstruation if there is gastric trouble, Nux Vomica is a sure remedy.

On the skin, elevated red patches of urticaria appear and the skin, particularly that of the face, burns hot. Yet the patient feels chilly the moment he moves or uncovers the body. At the same time he does not allow being covered. He is irritable, sullen and faultfinding.

For any type of fever where the above condition is present, Nux Vomica would be indicated. The fever may be inflammatory, periodic or it may be caused by a sore throat, by rheumatism or by any other disorder. Gastric symptoms would be present. Spasm with rigor and blueness of fingernails might come in the morning.

Nux Vomica acts best when administered at night. Gives response of body and mind. Of course, its use at other times is effective too.

The patient is better : From undisturbed nap, in the evening while at rest, by strong pressure, in damp, wet weather.

The patient is worse : By mental exertion, anger, touch, Waking up in the morning, After meals, By use of intoxicants, spices, narcotics, In dry cold weather.

❏❏❏

CHAPTER 77

Phosphoricum Acidum

The common acid "debility" is very marked in this remedy, producing a nervous exhaustion. Mental debility first, later physical. A congenital soil for the action of Phos. Acid is found in young people who grow rapidly, and who are overtaxed, mentally or physically. It is useful when the body is exposed to acute diseases, excesses grief, loss of vital fluids. Useful in relieving pain of cancer.

An excellent use of phosphoric Acidum is made in curing mental and physical debility and in acute and chronic diseases where the patient is tired in mind and body. The mental debility is a result of nervous exhaustion in persons who have been working overtime at a young age. Physical debility comes as a result of acute disease, sexual excesses, grief, and loss of vital fluids from the body. Haemorrhages in typhoid, therefore require Phosphoric Acidum.

According to Dr. J.T. Kent, mental symptoms are the first to develop in Phosphoric Acid. The remedy runs from the mental to the physical, from the brain to the muscles. Initially, the patient may forget names even of the members of his family or physical exertion. But soon the weakness in the muscles follows.

The Phosphoric Acid patient is apathetic, indifferent and confused. He has a cursing pain in the temples, worse on shaking or by noise. He feels a pressure on the top of the head and has vertigo towards evening, when standing or walking. His hair turns thin, grays early and falls out. Physical debility brings blue rings around eyes. The eyelids are inflamed and cold, the pupils dilated and with a glassy appearance. In the eyeballs there is pain as if they are forcibly pressed together and into the head.

The Phosphoric Acid patient has vertigo while lying in the bed. It is due to overall weakness of the mind and the body. The patient feels as if he is floating while lying in the bed. It is vertigo with ringing in the ears and with glassy eyes. The headaches of Phosphoric Acid are associated with mental weakness, brain fag; these come because the sufferer is so tired and exhausted.

Headache of growing students: Phosphoric Acid is a remedy for the headaches of students, especially of those who are growing too fast.

Blue rings around. Lids inflamed and cold. Pupils dilated. Glassy appearance. Averse to sunlight; sees colours as if a rainbow. Feel too large. Pain as if eyeballs were forcibly pressed together and into head.

The Phosphoric Acid patient has great physical weakness; he is too tired in the back, so tired in the muscles, so tired all over, a paralytic weakness. Ailments, which come from business cares; prolonged grief; young women suffering from unrequited affection or from loss of a loved one. Ailments resulting from care, grief, sorrow, chagrin, and homesickness. With drowsiness; night sweats towards morning; cold sweat down the back; cold sweats on the arms and hands more than on the feet; cold extremities; feeble circulation; feeble heart; withered face, catches cold on the slightest provocation.

In males, there is impotence; aversion to coition; loss of sexual desire; no erection. The penis becomes relaxed in the midst of an embrace and he cannot finish the act.

Phosphoric Acidum helps in herpes of the prepuce, in the oedema of the glans penis and swelling.

Phosphoric Acidum is useful in diabetes where the urine is frequent, profuse and milky. At night the frequency increases. The passing of urine is preceded by anxiety and is followed by burning.

Debility, which needs Phosphoric Acidum, also causes cramps in the upper arms and the wrists. At night there are pains as if the bones were scraped.

According to Dr. E. B. Nash, Phosphoric Acidum is one of the best remedies in typhoid fever where the patient lies in a stupor, unconscious of all that is going on around him, but, when aroused, is fully conscious. He has a crushing pain on the vertex, a pin in the occiput or nape of the neck and appears physically weak or exhausted, wants to lie down, does not want company or to be noticed or spoken to.

In advanced typhoid when there is prostration distension in the abdomen, a dry, brown tongue, glassy eyes, gradually approaching unconsciousness, a little thirst increasing to intense thirst, a desire to be left alone, bleeding from the nose, lungs, bowels, sunken eyes, discolored lips gradually becoming very black, Phosphoric Acidum is indicated. It checks the haemorrhage, causes a rally and prevents dropsy.

In Phosphoric Acid, there is an amelioration of complaints by their ending in diarrhoea. The diarrhoea is copious, thin and watery, whitish grey and the patient feels thereafter comfortable, free and happy. He is worse if the diarrhoea slackens.

Podophyllum is indicated where the stool is copious thin, offensive and has a horrible stench. The stool is painless in both Podophyllum and Phosphoric Acid does not have the great prostration of Podophyllum. Its stool is whitish-grey like dirty white paint while in Podophyllum it is yellow.

Urine is frequent, profuse, watery, and milky. Diabetes. Micturition proceeded by anxiety and followed by burning. Frequent urination at night. Phosphaturia.

Recommended potency: 30, 200.

The patient is better from keeping warm, from diarrhoea.

The patient is worse from exertion, being talked to, loss of vital fluids and sexual excesses.

❑❑❑

CHAPTER 78

Phosphorus

Phosphorus irritates, inflames and degenerates mucous membranes, irritates, and inflames serous membranes, inflames spinal cord and nerves, causing paralysis, destroys bone, especially the lower jaw and tibia; disorganizes the blood, causing fatty degeneration of blood vessels and every tissue and organs of the body and thus gives rise to haemorrhages.

Produces a picture of destructive metabolism. Causes yellow atrophy of the liver and sub-acute hepatitis. Tall, slender persons, narrow chested, with thin, transparent skin, weakened by loss of animal fluids, with great nervous debility, emaciation seems to be under the special influence of Phosphorus. Great susceptibility to external impressions, to light, sound, odors, touch, thunderstorms. Polycythaemia, fatty degeneration, cirrhosis, and caries are pathological states calling for this remedy, inflammations of the respiratory tract. Paralytic symptoms. Ill effects of iodine and excessive use of salt, worse lying on left side.

The first indication for Phosphorus is given by an intense sensation of burning in various parts of the body like the mouth, the lungs, the stomach, the small intestines, the anus, up the spine, the palm of the hand, and even the face. The patient craves for cold food, but this food is vomited as soon as it reaches the stomach. There is an insatiable hunger, an empty gone feeling in the stomach, in the whole abdomen.

Even the smallest of wounds bleed easily. The wounds heal but break out again.

A feeling of intense heat running up the back or between the scapulae is relieved by Phosphorus. There is burning of the hands (Sulphur is indicated for burning of the feet)

There are men and women in whom the sexual appetite is insatiable. This leads them into a mania in which they expose themselves, take off their clothes in public. Such maniacs are not good for physical sex because the mania is succeeded by extreme impotence. Phosphorus is the remedy in such cases.

When the patient fears to be left alone, is afraid of the dark, is restless and suffers from great anxiety, Phosphorus helps.

Phosphorus is required for acute hepatitis, for fatty degeneration of the liver, for jaundice, for cirrhosis, pancreatic diseases and for large yellow spots on the abdomen.

Phosphorus is indicated for spasmodic stricture of the oesophagus. There is an inability to swallow food. Whatever is swallowed comes out immediately, as if there is a pressure working upwards.

Think of Phosphorus in cases of profuse diarrhoea when the stool pours out as from a municipal hydrant without a washer. At the same time, this is also a remedy in cases of constipation where the faeces are dry, hard, and long and are expelled with great difficulty.

The lower as well as the upper eyelids swell and so does the whole face. Phosphorus is required.

In chronic running nose accompanied by haemorrhage, Phosphorus is indicated. The handkerchief of the patient is always bloody. Phosphorus takes care of easily bleeding polyps.

Phosphorus is the medicine for persistently bleeding gums after tooth extraction. It is better to go to the dentist for extraction after taking a dose of Arnica 200, to be followed by Phosphorus 200 after the surgery. Later when bleeding has been controlled. Arnica should be continued. Phosphorus can be repeated if the bleeding has not stopped.

Necrosis of the jawbone and of the tibia requires Phosphorus.

Phosphorus is indicated in cases where the patient is better if he can get some sleep. (Where the problems are similar, but the patient is worse after sleep, Lachesis is indicated.) The patient would be in stupor and would mutter in delirium in a low voice.

In typhoid when there is a lung complication, Phosphorus is the remedy.

Phosphorus is the remedy in the following as well.

i. Dandruff, the falling out of hair in large bunches, itching of the scalp.

ii. Black floaters before the eyes, green halo about light. Letters appear red. Pain in the orbital bones. Thrombosis of the retinal vessels.

iii. Tearing pain in facial bones.

iv. Severe pain in the larynx. On that account, difficulty in speech. Great hoarseness.

v. Sensory and motor paralysis ascending from ends of fingers and toes. Great difficulty in the hand. Stitching pain in elbow and shoulder joints. Numbness in arms and hands.

Recommended potency : 200,1000 in cholera.

Generally used as an acute remedy.

The patient is worse: Early morning, in hot weather, during dentition.

□□□

CHAPTER 79

Pulsatilla Nigricans

The word *PULSATILLA* is derived from *PULSATUS* meaning to beat or to strike as it pulsates from the blowing winds.

The weathercock among remedies. The disposition and mental state are the chief guiding symptoms to the selection of Pulsatilla. It is pre-eminently a female remedy, especially for mild, gentle, yielding disposition. Sad crying readily; weeps when talking; changeable, contradictory. The patient seeks the open air; always feels better there, even though he is chilly. Mucous membranes are all affected. Discharges thick, bland, and yellowish green. Often indicated after abuse of Iron tonics, and after badly- managed measeals. Symptoms ever changing. Thirstless, peevish and chilly. When first serious impairment of health is referred to age of puberty. Great sensitiveness.

Pulsatilla cures chronic colds, fatty dyspepsia, and painful and scanty menstruation. One of the leading indications for the use of Pulsatilla is a thick, bland, yellowish or green discharge from mucous membranes in the body. Such discharges are to be found in nasal catarrh, in expectoration from the ears, the eyes, the lungs, ulcers, leucorrhoea and in gonorrhoea. In most such cases Pulsatilla leads to a cure. In the vagina, however, this discharge is excoriating and not bland.

An important indication leading us to Pulsatilla is that pain in the body travels from one part to another, from one joint to another. Haemorrhage occurs, stops and occurs again. The patient passes different types of stool. Thus in every problem there is a changeability of symptoms. This occurs in rheumatism, neuralgic pain, in old colds, in cholera of infants, in hot weather and so on.

The pulsatilla patient is of a mild, yielding disposition. She is thirstless, peevish and chilly. She wants her head high on pillows and lies with her hands above the head.

There is nothing like Pulsatilla in curing sinus where yellowish, green, bland mucus is flowing outwards. The nose is ever stuffed. It may be necessary to administer four doses of Pastille 30 everyday for a week or more to completely eliminate this cold. In all such cases, it would be noticed that the patient has lost his sense of smell. After a few days of the treatment, he would be able to enjoy even the mild fragrance of a red rose. (In Kali Bi, the yellowish, green discharge in chronic cold virtually hardens into a rope and drips into the throat. It is very difficult to take out. That distinguishes its use from that of Pulsatilla where the discharge comes out easily.)

Next to its importance in the treatment of chronic, bad old colds, pulsatilla is greatly effective in cases where a patient gets easy indigestion on account of his fondness for fats, heavy food, pastries, cakes, fruit, creamy food and rich food of any type. There is flatulence, pain in the stomach an hour or so after a meal. In most such cases, there is a loss of taste. Lack of thirst is another indication of Pulsatilla. Along with taste, the smell would have been lost. A dry mouth, no thirst, lack of taste and loss of smell are important indications for the use of Pulsatilla.

An interesting cure achieved by Pulsatilla is in the case of troublesome, chronic constipation. In such cases, the stool is large, hard and difficult to excrete. No two motions are alike. Blind haemorrhoids with a violent may accompany such constipation, stitching pain. Dysentery and diarrhoea alternate.

For thick, bland, yellowish or green discharge of pus from the ears, Pulsatilla is a sure cure. The discharge smells foul. The pain is worse at night. The acuteness of the hearing is affected.

The same is true of eyes where the lids are inflamed, glued together on account of a greenish, yellowish and thick discharge coming in profusion.

Pulsatilla is a cure for styes on the eyelids.

Pulsatilla is a remedy in varicose veins bleed black blood, which easily coagulates.

Pulsatilla is an excellent remedy in cases of suppressed or scanty, late and painful menstruation. The patient is restless and does not get relief even by tossing in the bed. The menses start, stop, start and flow, stop again. The patient is usually of a mild, gentle and sweet temperament. She may be easily lead to shed tears and is quite touchy over anything. Pulsatilla is also an effective remedy in cases of abnormally delayed menstruation in young ladies of mild, gentle, and tearful temperament.

Pulsatilla relieves headache-accompanying menstruation. The headache is usually throbbing and congestive. Pulsatilla also relieves headache coming from overeating or from taking rich food.

In women, Pulsatilla cures nymphomania. Sexual desire is beyond limits and is uncontrollable. Pulsatilla also takes care of thick, yellow, green and excoriating leucorrhoea. The vagina is raw in such cases.

In men, Pulsatilla helps in orchitis, inflammation and the swelling of the testicles from mumps and from catching cold. The patient has strong sexual desire, long lasting, morning erections. Gonorrhoea with thick, yellow or green discharge requires Pulsatilla. In acute prostatitis, Pulsatilla is indicated.

Recommended potency: 30,200.

The patient is better : By taking cold food and drinks, though not thirsty, By cold application, By slow walking, in open, cool fresh air., With head raised on a pillow.

The patient is worse: By taking rich fat food, after eating; towards evening., in a warm room, by warm baths., Lying on left or painless side.

❑❑❑

CHAPTER 80

Rhus Toxicodendron

The word *RHUS* means red because its flowers and leaves are red in colour. *TOXICODENDRON* means poison tree.

The effects on the skin, rheumatic pains, mucous membrane affections, and a typhoid type of fever, make this remedy frequently indicated. It mainly affects fibrous tissues, joints, tendons, sheaths producing pain and stiffness. Ailments from strains, over lifting, getting wet while perspiring. Rheumatism in the cold season.

Rhus Tox is the first remedy one should think of in any muscular pain where the cutting pain and soreness are temporarily relieved by movement. This is in direct contrast to Bryonia where movement aggravates pain.

The patient is restless, internally uneasy, and nervous. He wants to be on the move because it temporarily relieves his discomfort. Restlessness is evident in Aconite and Arsenic Alb also but there change does not relieve discomfort.

The pain, which responds to Rhus Tox, is a tearing-asunder pain, a bruised pain often attended by numbness and paralysis of the limbs with loss of sensation. This pain comes in the night. The pain is quite often caused by exposure to the cold, particularly in wet weather, on exposure when perspiring.

Muscular lameness and stiffness is relieved by Rhus Tox, weather it is of a rheumatic character or whether it has been caused by a strain like the lifting heavy articles or unscientific, unguided and excessive muscular exercise. In sprains when Arnica has reduced the pain and swelling, if any, Rhus Tox should be administered to strengthen the person.

When the limbs are stiff and paralyzed there is tearing pain in the tendons, ligaments and membranes of joints. The joints are hot, painful and swollen. There is rheumatic pain in the nape of the neck, in the loins and in the thighs. There is tenderness in the knee-joint. In all such cases when there is temporary amelioration on movement, Rhus Tox does wonders. Rhus Tox is excellent for old chronic rheumatic conditions. And so it is paralysis of the arms, when on grasping anything a tingling and prickling sensation is left in the hands and the fingers.

Infantile paralysis caused by exposure in damp weather after perspiration, Rhus Tox comes handy.

In lumbago there is nothing to beat Rhus Tox and invariably it is indicated when there is temporary improvement in the condition of the patient on movement. He is better lying on a hard surface. Backache, even myelitis (pain in the spinal membranes) which has been caused by exposure, by lying in damp sheets, by getting soaked in sudden rain, while perspiring or by strain, responds very well to Rhus Tox.

Rhus Tox is of use in left-sided sciatica, tearing pain in the lower limbs, worse during rest and ameliorated from motion for a short while. This sciatica pain has been caused by catching a cold from damp and cold weather, from exposure and from suppression of sweat on exposure. Rhus Tox 1000 or 10000 helps greatly to relieve sciatica pain.

In influenza with body pain, Rhus Tox ranks with Gelesemium and Eupatorium Perf. There is tormenting, dry cough before and during chill.

Rhus Tox is a cure in dysentery where there is pain in the thighs and legs.

Rhus Tox is an excellent remedy in eczema of the face and of the genitals. The scrotum becomes thick and hard. There is swelling in the genitals. The itching is severe. In facial eczema, there is chronic suppuration and eruption. Rhus Tox is valuable for erysipelas of the vesicular variety. On the face there are large, burning blisters. Inflammation extends rapidly. The skin becomes purple and pits on the pressure. And so on in characteristic restlessness and an intense itching.

In the mouth the triangular tip of the tongue is red. The jaws crack when chewing.

Recommended potency: 200, 1000, 10000.

The patient is better from motion, walking, in warm, dry weather, by change of position, by warm application, bath, rubbing, on stretching out limbs.

The patient is worse in cold, wet, rainy weather, during sleep, at night, on being drenched while perspiring, in cold fresh air, which is so intolerable that, it makes the skin painful.

□□□

CHAPTER 81

Secale Cornutum

It produces contraction of the unstriped muscular fibers, hence a constringent feeling throughout the whole body. This produces an anemic condition, coldness, numbness, mortification and gangrene. A useful remedy for old persons with shriveled skin- thin, scrawny old women. All the Secale conditions are better from cold; the whole body is pervaded by great heat. Haemorrhages continued oozing, thin, fetid, watery black blood. Debility, anxiety, emaciation, though appetite and thirst may be excessive. Facial and abdominal muscles twitch. Secale lowers the flow of pancreatic juice by raising the blood pressure.

Menstrual colic, with coldness and intolerance of heat. Passive haemorrhages in feeble, cachetic women. Burning pains in uterus, brownish, offensive leucorrhoea. Menses irregular, copious, dark, continuous oozing of watery blood until next period. Threatened abortion about the third month. During labor no expulsive action, though everything is relaxed. After-pains. Suppression of milk; breasts do not fill properly. Dark, offensive lochia. Puerperal fever, putrid discharges, tympanitis, coldness, suppressed urine.

Cholera-like stools, with coldness and cramps. Olive-green, thin, putrid, bloody, with icy coldness and intolerance of being covered, with great exhaustion. Involuntary stools; no sensation of passing faces, anus wide open. Unnatural ravenous appetite; craves acids. Thirst unquenchable. Burning in stomach and abdomen; tympanites. Eructation of bad odor. Tongue dry, cracked; blood like ink exudes, coated thick; viscid, yellowish, cold livid. Tingling of tip of tongue, which is stiff. Tongue swollen, paralyzed.

Paralysis of bladder. Retention, with unsuccessful urging. Discharge of black blood from bladder. Enuresis in old people.

Shriveled, numb; mottled dusky-blue tinge. Raynaud's disease. Blue color, Dry gangrene, developing slowly. Varicose ulcers. Burning sensation; better by cold; wants parts uncovered, though cold to touch. Formication; petechiae. Slight wounds continue to bleed. Livid sports. Boils, small, painful, with green contents; mature slowly. Skin feels cold to touch; yet covering is not tolerated. Great aversion to heat. Formication under skin.

This remedy produces a progressive general anaemia. It is shown by the peculiar cachexia of anaemia, pale, bloodless, jaundiced color. By its effect on the blood corpuscles it produces a general anaemia, threatening not only the life of a part, but vitiating the whole life of the bodily economy. It is a sort of a mechanical anaemia.

Cold, dry hands and feet of excessive smokers with feeling of fuzziness in fingers. Trembling, staggering gait. Formication, pain and spasmodic movements. Numbness. Fingers and feet bluish, shriveled, spread apart or bent backwards, numb Violent cramps. Icy coldness of extremities. Violent pain in fingertips, tingling in toes.

Suits the stage of collapse with desire to keep cool; cholera infantum with profuse undigested stools, watery and offensive, followed by prostration; the movements are copious and come in spurts; the skin is wrinkled, dry and cold; patient is almost pulse less, cold, but averse to being covered, spasmodic twitching of muscles, spreads fingers apart, eyes sunken, features pinched, are important indicating symptoms of Secale.

Spinal irritation, tingling of lower extremities; can bear only slightest covering. Locomotor ataxia. Formation and numbness. Myelitis. Secale is recommended for sudden and rapidly recurring convulsions, with rapid sinking of strength and paralysis of the spinal nerves. This remedy produces a condition very similar to locomotor ataxia. It has in the first place three of the principle symptoms of the disease, namely:

1. Absence of knee jerk.
2. Fulgurating pains.
3. Ataxia.

Contraction of lower limbs, on account of which the patient staggers. Inability to govern the movements.

Trembling of limbs, sometimes with pains.

Formication of hands and feet. Numbness of extremities.

Excessive sensation of heat with aversion to being covered.

These are all symptoms found in patients and Secale will be the remedy when these are present.

This remedy corresponds to passive, painless, dark, offensive haemorrhages in thin scrawny women with formication and tingling in the limbs, surface of body cold and desire to be uncovered. It is characterized by slow oozing, dark, thin and persistent and worse from motion.

Pupils dilated. Incipient cataract, senile especially in women. Eyes sunken and surrounded by a blue margin.

Face is pale, pinched, and sunken. Cramps commence in face and spread over whole body. Livid spots on face. Spasmodic distortion.

Sleep is profound and long. Insomnia with restlessness, fever, anxious dreams. Insomnia of drug and liquor habitués.

Recommended potency: 30

Patient is better from cold, uncovering, rubbing, and stretching out limbs.

Patient is worse from heat and warm covering.

❑❑❑

CHAPTER 82

Sepia

Acts especially on the portal system, with venous congestion. Stasis and thereby ptosis of viscera and weariness and misery. Weakness, yellow complexion, bearing-down sensation, especially in women, upon whose organism it has most pronounced effect. Pains extend down to back, chills easily. Tendency to abortion. Hot flashes at menopause with weakness and perspiration. Upward tendency of its symptoms. Easy fainting,' Ball' sensation in inner parts. Sepia acts best on brunettes. All pains are from below up. One of the most important uterine remedies. Tubercular patients with chronic hepatic troubles and uterine reflexes. Feels cold even in warm room.

The most important indications of Sepia are in the problems of women relating to the uterus. It has been called the best uterine remedy available. The patient feels that all her internal organs would come out of the pelvic region. She has to sit with legs crossed to relieve this feeling. Sepia is a chronic remedy. It can take care of long standing problems.

Pelvic displacement, with inflammation, ulceration, leucorrhoea and even malignant growth would be alleviated by Sepia. It is of great help in prolapse of the uterus and of the vagina.

Sepia is the medicine when the vagina is painful, especially on intercourse.

There is weakness in the small of the back. The pain extends from the pelvic region into the back. Sepia is needed.

Yellow, greenish leucorrhoea with intense itching indicates Sepia. Menstruation is irregular. It is either too late or scanty, or too early and profuse. In either circumstance, there is sharp pain, upwards in the vagina.

Sepia is indicated in ulceration of the cervix. Its use is more effective than any local application.

With the stoppage of menstruation, women suffer from flushes of heat, perspiration and faintness. At the same time, there is a feeling of bearing down as if every thing would escape through the vagina. Such cases require Sepia. (In case the symptoms are accompanied by a burning sensation, Sulphur is indicated.)

Women suffering from the aforesaid problems might also have hemicrania, that is, headache on one side of the head. The pain comes in terrible shocks. Uncontrollable. The patient has persistent jerks of the head. Sepia is required.

Emotionally a Sepia patient is unable to feel natural love, to be affectionate. She permits no opposition to her opinions. Her problems are aggravated by noise. She is indolent, sad, indifferent and easily offended.

Sepia is a remedy for the exhausted housewife, overburdened with work and children. She is harassed. It helps maid sitting on haunches and working hard, bending over their laundry, harassed by weeping brats.

The Sepia patient is very weak. A short walk tires her. She faints easily from extremes of cold or heat, from riding, from kneeling and what not. She cannot work hard. She feels cold even in the warm room.

Yellow blotches are noticed on the face of the Sepia patient, a saddle like yellow distribution of brown, yellow spots on the nose and cheeks. The face is pale and sullen.

In chronic cold with inflammation where there is a thick, greenish and bland discharge with thick plugs and crusts. Sepia is indicated. In such cases, even if there were a postnasal discharge of lumpy mucus, Sepia would be great remedy.

Sepia helps in a prolapse of the rectum along with pelvic congestion. There is a sensation of a ball. There is a constant oozing of moisture from the anus.

Infantile diarrhoea, worse from boiled milk, is controlled by Sepia.

Sepia relieves obstinate constipation where the stool has to be physically removed. It happens mostly in children.

A characteristic of Sepia discharge, whether in the back of the throat, from the nasal passages or from the vagina, is its being excoriating and milky leucorrhoea at times take the appearance of curds, thick, cheesy and horribly offensive. Some times, this discharge is thick, green and yellow.

Sepia is indicated in chronic cases.

Lachesis is inimical to Sepia.

The patient is better : By exercise, by pressure, in warmth of bed, by hot application, Sitting crossed legged, Loosing clothes, after sleep.

The patient is worse : In the forenoon, in the evening, By washing, laundry, exertion, Jar, Walking, In damp cold air, At climacteric, Taking milk, Left side.

□□□

CHAPTER 83

Silicea

Imperfect assimilation and consequent defective nutrition, it goes further and produces neurasthenic states in consequence, and increased susceptibility to nervous stimuli and exaggerated reflexes. Diseases of bones, caries and necrosis. In TB it must be used with care, for here it may cause the absorption of scar tissue, liberate the disease, walled in, to new activities. It is a deep acting remedy and slow in action. It is meant for scrofulous children with large head, open fontanels and sutures, distended abdomen, slow in walking. Ill effects of vaccination. It is related to all fistulous openings. Ripens abscesses since it promotes suppuration.

Silica patient is cold, chilly, hugs the fire, wants plenty warm clothing, and hates drafts, hands and feet cold, worse in winter. Lack of vital heat. Prostration of mind and body. Great sensitiveness to taking cold. Intolerance of alcoholic stimulants. Ailments attended with pus formation.

In inflammation with pus formation, which has become chronic, silicea is of great help. It is equally useful in grandular or bony ulceration. Think of silicea in whitlow, unhealthy skin, smelly feet, mammary abscess, mammary cancer, TB of the skin, the bone or of the abdomen,

Deep-seated pus formation, even in tendons and ligaments, responds to silicea very well.

Silicea helps in the expulsion of the foreign bodies from tissues because of its power to take care of deep-rooted abscesses. It helps in abscesses, boils, and old fistulous ulcers. Breaks down scar tissue.

In case Hepar Sulph has discharged pus already formed, silicea would heal that part of the body after the discharge. (In wounds that refuse to heal gunpowder 30 or 200 is required).

The silicea patient is weak and has lax muscles. He is sensitive to cold air, takes cold easily, especially when his head or foot is uncovered. His face is pale, his skin fine. He is nervous and irritable, lacks grit. He lacks stamina. He dreads failure. He has profuse sweat on the head and offensive sweat on the feet. Pain in the head begins at occiput, and spreads overhead and settles over eyes. Vertigo from looking up better by wrapping up warmly, when lying on left side.

With silicea, as Dr. Nash puts it, the patient's spirits rise, hope revives, the weakness and depression give way to a feeling of returning strength and health.

A very important sphere of influence of silicea is in cases of patients who can never get rid of their cold. There is violent cough when lying down. The sputum they take out is constantly full of mucus and is offensive. It is thick, yellow and lumpy. Here silicea should be thought of as a chronic of Pulsatilla.

Silicea helps in old cases of catarrh of the ear where there is offensive, thick and yellow discharge. There is roaring in the ears, a hissing like that of steam.

When the tonsils are swollen after a cold and there is pain as if a pin is pricking. Silicea should be thought of as a remedy.

Silicea is of great use in constipation. The rectum is weak, paralysed. The stool protrudes and then slips back. This constipation is quite typical to teething children. The rectum appears to have lost its expulsive power.

Silicea helps in old anal fistula, in haemorrhoids with fissures which are painful and where there is a spasm of the sphincter.

Serous cysts in the vagina, projecting out or upwards, of the size of a pea need silicea.

Silicea gives relief in warty growths on the skin, moist eruptions, pimples, pustules, abscesses, and suppurating cavities.

Crippled nails, nails with white spots need silicea.

Weak children whose assimilation is defective, although food intake is sufficient, with shrunken limbs, pinched face, pick up after administration of Silicea. Such a child has a big belly.

" Silicea is a chronic of Pulsatilla and is its complementary. It is Puls, only more so, a deeper, more profound remedy".: Dr. Kent.

Mercury and Silicea do not follow each other well.

Recommended potency: 200 and higher.

The patient is better : In wet and humid weather, in summer, by warmth, Wrapping up head.

The patient is worse : Taking down, Lying down, Getting feet wet, Uncovering the head, At new moon, Washing, In damp cold.

□□□

CHAPTER 84

Sulphur

This is a great Hahnemannian anti- psoric. Its action is centrifugal - from within outward - having an elective affinity for the skin, where it produces heat and burning, with itching; made worse by heat of bed. Inertia and relaxation of fibre; hence feebleness of tone chracterizes its symptoms. Ebullitions of heat, dislike of water, dry and hard hair and skin, red orifices, sinking feeling at stomach about 11.00am, cat-nap sleep; always indicate sulphur homoeopathically. Standing is the worst position for sulphur patients it is always uncomfortable. Dirty, filthy people, prone to skin affections. Aversion to being washed. When carefully selected remedies fail to act, especially in acute diseases, it frequently arouses the reactionary powers of the organism. Complaints that relapse. General offensive character of discharge and exhalations. Very red lips and face, flushing easily. Often use in beginning the treatment of chronic cases and in finishing acute ones.

Think of Sulphur whenever there is a burning sensation. The burning may be inside the head or on the scalp, a burning mucus from the nose, a burning in the face with redness, a burning in the mouth, on the tongue, a burning sore throat which is dry, a burning in the stomach, a burning and pressure in the rectum, a burning and itching in piles which come in bunches, a burning while passing urine, a burning in the vagina or nipples burning like fire, a burning in the hands, in the feet, on the skin, a burning in the soles of the feet and the palms of the hands, and so on. In all such cases, Sulphur gives instant relief. (For the sensation of coldness, Calcarea Carb is indicated.)

Here it would be advisable to distinguish the burning indication in another medicine, that is Arsenic Alb. in acute sickness, that is, a sickness which is recent and which runs a short course, we use Arsenic Alb. as against Sulphur is used in chronic problems.

In skin problems, the best use of Sulphur is made where burning follows scratching. There are itching eruptions on the skin everywhere. The sequence of the problem would be starting with voluptuous itching, relieved by scratching and followed by burning.

A very interesting feature has been noted in certain patients with skin problems. They have a dry, scaly and unhealthy skin. They do not like washing and are, therefore, filthy. Washing even aggravates their problems. There is a sweating excoriation especially in corners like the armpits and the leg pits. The hands are hot and sweating. In all such cases, Sulphur is indicated.

The human body has many orifices, like the mouth, the ears, the eyelids, the urethra, the anus etc. these orifices become red like vermilion. There is itching and burning. Sulphur helps remarkably in such cases.

Induration from pressure, like corns, callosities in the sides, gets relief by use of Sulphur.

Sulphur cures the susceptibility to catch cold. A person may take a bath or he may get over-heated. He may enter a cold room or might over-exert. A change of weather occurs. Whatever be the reason, the patient catches a cold, and his nose starts running. Sulphur would take care of this tendency. Administer one dose of Sulphur 200, early morning, once a week for 2 months.

Sulphur does good to persons who lead s sedentary life, confined to their rooms in study or in meditation or who take almost no exercise, take simple food which is not even nourishing and look lean, lank and hungry. Dr. Hering has called a Sulphur patient " A ragged philosopher ". For him, chilliness is absolutely irrelevant. He is filthy, his odour is foul; his discharges are excoriating.

In men if the prepuce is narrow and difficult to pull back, sulphur helps. When an erection does not occur even though the desire is strong. The mind is willing, the body is not. Discharge occurs on contact.

For women whose periods are too late, short, scanty and painful, Sulphur is the remedy. The blood is thick, black and excoriating. In between, there is burning and acrid leucorrhoea. The nipples are cracked and burn. There is severe itching on the vulva. Burning in the vagina.

Sulphur occupies a very prominent place in the homoeopathic materia medica. It has been found after extensive research that when seemingly indicated remedies do not cure, particularly in acute cases, Sulphur should be thought of. Sulphur brings out the curing properties of a medicine, which has already been administered, and hence it is useful when given as an intermittent remedy say, one dose a week when a particular treatment takes more than a few weeks. Thus, it helps in complaints, which relapses.

In such cases it would be useful to administer Sulphur early in the morning. Ten pills should be dissolved in half a teacup of luke warm water and the solution sipped slowly over 30 minutes. The medicine should not be allowed to stay in the mouth and rolled on the tongue for a minute after every sip.

Sulphur is very effective in chronic constipation as an intermittent remedy.

Complaints in which Sulphur is a remedy come on from the warmth of the bed and, therefore, quite a few of these problems arise at night. The Sulphur patient is disturbed by a change in temperature. Bathing aggravates the problem and so does standing for a long time. His headache comes after an evening meal. He drinks much and eats little.

If an infant does not develop properly, if his bones do not grow, use Calcarea Carb followed by Sulphur.

In acute problems Sulphur follows Aconite very well. Merc Sol and Calcarea Carb are useful after Sulphur and not before in chronic problems.

Sulphur is used in the beginning of treatment in chronic cases. In acute cases, it is used to give a finishing touch.

Recommended potency: 200 and higher.

The patient is better from dry, warm weather, drawing up affected limbs, lying on right side, from open windows when respiration is difficult.

The patient is worse in the morning, 11 a.m., washing, bathing, at rest, when standing, at night, from alcoholic drinks, periodically.

❑❑❑

Glossary

ACIDITY-Excessive acid quality, as of the gastric juice.

ACRID - biting, sharp to taste or smell.

ADENOIDS- Characterized by debility, low blood pressure and a brownish skin discoloration.

ALVEOLI- Air sacs in the lungs.

AMENORRHEA - Abnormal suppression or absence of menstruation.

ANEMIA - Lack of red blood corpuscles.

ANAESTHESIA - Loss of sensation induced by anesthetics.

ANEURYSMS - A sac formed by dilatation of a blood vessel.

ANGUISH - Agonizing physical or mental pain.

APHONIA - Loss of speech, or voicelessness.

APHTHAE - Small ulcers, especially the whitish or reddish spots in the mouth.

APPENDICITIS - Inflammation of the Vermiform Appendix.

APPETITE - A desire for food or drink.

ARTHRITIS - Inflammation of the joint.

ATONY - Lack of sufficient muscular tone or strength.

ATROPHY - The wasting away of tissues, organs or the entire body.

BACKACHE - A pain especially in the lumber region of the back.

BILE - A liver secretion, bitter, alkaline, brownish-yellow or greenish- yellow, stored in the gallbladder, and discharged into the duodenum to help digestion.

BILIRUBIN - A reddish-yellow organic compound derived from haemoglobin during normal destruction of erythrocytes blood cells containing haemoglobin.

BRADYCARDIA - Abnormally slow heartbeat, less than 60 beats per minute.

BRUISE - An injury on the surface of unbroken skin, due to haemorrhage into tissue from ruptured vessels.

CALLOSITY - Hardened skin due to pressure with loss of sensitivity.

CARBUNCLE - Severe abscess.

CARCINOMA - Cancerous ulcer.

CERVICITIS - Inflammation of the cervix, of the uterus.

CHEILOSIS - Cracking and dryness of the lip surface and of the angles of the mouth.

CHOREA - A nervous disorder, especially of children, characterized by uncontrollable and irregular movements of the muscles of the arms, legs and face.

COLIC - Acute, sudden, violent fit of pain caused by spasms, obstruction or distention in the abdomen.

CONCUSSION - Violent shaking or shock to a soft structure, especially of the brain.

CONDYLOMA - A wart like excrescence on the skin, usually in the region of the anus and genitals.

CONTAGIOUS - Catching, transmissible by direct or indirect contact.

CONVALESCENCE - Process of regaining health.

COPIOUS - Plentiful, abundant.

CRAMPS - Severe pain causing sudden .voluntary muscular contraction, often occurring in the leg or shoulder as a result of strain or chill.

CYANOSIS - A bluish discoloration of the skin.

CYST - Abnormal sac of fluid on or in the body.

DEGLUTITION - The process or act of swallowing.

DELIRIUM - Disordered state of mind, especially during fever.

DISTENSION - Bloated or turgid form as if from internal pressure.

EMACIATED - Thin from illness or starvation.

EMPHYSEMA - Abnormal distension of a part of the body particularly the lungs.

ENURESIS - Involuntary urination.

EPILEPSY - Disorder of the nervous system, causing fits.

EVACUATION - To excrete or discharge waste matter from the bowels.

EXPECTORATION - Cough and spitting of phlegm.

FISSURE - A groove or furrow in skin.

FLATULENCE - Presence of gas in the digestive tract.

GANGRENE - Decay of body tissue, due to failure in blood supply injury or disease.

HAEMORRHOIDS - Varicose veins at or near the anus.

HALLUCINATION - Illusion of seeing or hearing something not actually present.

HEARTBURN - Burning sensation in the lower part of the chest.

HERNIA - Protrusion of a portion of an organ through an abnormal opening.

HICCUPS - Cough- like stooping of breath.

HYDROCELE - Accumulation of serous fluid in a bodily cavity, especially the testes.

IMPOTENCY - Inability to copulate successfully or procreate.

INDIGNATION - Anger roused by something unjust or wicked.

INSOMNIA - Chronic sleeplessness.

KERATITIS - Inflammation of the cornea.

LANCINATING - Like the piercing of a lance.

LOQUACITY - Tendency to talk much.

MASTITIS - Inflammation of the breasts.

MENOPAUSE - Time of life when a woman ceases to menstruate.

MENNORRHAGIA - Abnormally heavy menstrual flow.

METRORRHAGIA - Irregular uterine bleeding, of normal amount but of longer duration.

MUCOPURULENT - Infected and full of mucus.

NECROSIS - The pathologic death of living tissue in an animal.

NEURALGIA - Sharp pain along a nerve.

OEDEMA - An excessive accumulation of serous fluid in the tissues.

ORCHITIS - Inflammation of the testes.

OSTEOMYELITIS - Inflammation of the bone marrow.

OTORRHOEA - A discharge from the ear.

PALPITATION - Rapid throbbing.

PALSY - Paralysis especially with involuntary tremors.

PHIMOSIS - Constriction of the orifice of the prepuce so that it cannot be drawn back over the glans.

PLEURISY - Inflammation of the pleura.

POLYP - A growth protruding from the mucous lining of an organ, such as the nose.

PROLAPSE - The slipping forward and down, out of place, of an organ in the body.

PYORRHOEA - Inflammation of the gum and tooth socket.

RETCHING - Straining one's throat as of vomiting.

SCLEROSIS - Abnormal hardening of the tissue.

SOMNAMBULAMCE - State of walking in one's sleep.

SPONDYLOSIS - Vertebral immobility and fusion of a joint due to disease, injury or surgery.

SQUINT - Have one eye turned abnormally from the line of gaze of the other.

STOMATITIS - Inflammation of the mucous tissue of the mouth.

STRANGURY - Slow, painful urination witı. spasms of the urethra and bladder.

TACHYCARDIA - Abnormally rapid heart beat.

THROMBOSIS - Formation of a clot of blood in a blood vessel or organ of the body.

TWITCHING - Pulling with a slight jerk, quivering or contracting spasmodically.

URETHRITIS - Inflammation of the urethra.

VAGINISMUS - A painful spasm of the vagina.

VARICOSE VEINS - Permanently swollen veins.

VESICLES - Small hollow structure in the body.

WARTS - Small, hard, abnormal growth on skin.

WHEEZING - Breathing with a horse whistling sound.

WHITLOW - Small abscess under or affecting a nail.